# Chromosome Anomalies and
# Prenatal Development: An Atlas

# OXFORD MONOGRAPHS ON MEDICAL GENETICS

## General Editors

ARNO G. MOTULSKY     MARTIN BOBROW
PETER S. HARPER     CHARLES SCRIVER

## Former Editors

J. A. FRASER ROBERTS     C. O. CARTER

OXFORD MONOGRAPHS ON MEDICAL GENETICS NO. 21

# Chromosome Anomalies and Prenatal Development: An Atlas

DOROTHY WARBURTON

JULIANNE BYRNE

NINA CANKI

NEW YORK · OXFORD    OXFORD UNIVERSITY PRESS · 1991

Oxford University Press

Oxford   New York   Toronto
Delhi   Bombay   Calcutta   Madras   Karachi
Petaling Jaya   Singapore   Hong Kong   Tokyo
Nairobi   Dar es Salaam   Cape Town
Melbourne   Auckland

and associated companies in
Berlin   Ibadan

Warburton, Dorothy.
Chromosome Anomalies and Prenatal Development: An Atlas
by Dorothy Warburton, Julianne Byrne, Nina Canki.
p.   cm.—(Oxford monographs on medical genetics ; no. 21)
Includes bibliographical references.
ISBN 0-19-505145-9
1. Fetus—Abnormalities—Atlases.   2. Human chromosome
abnormalities—Atlases.   3. Miscarriage—Atlases.   I. Byrne,
Julianne M.   II. Canki, Nina.   III. Title.   IV. Series.
[DNLM: 1. Abortion—genetics—atlases.   2. Chromosome Aberrations—
atlases.   3. Fetal Development—atlases.   WQ 17 W254a]
RG627.W296   1990      618.3' 2043—dc20
DNLM/DLC for Library of Congress          90-7606

2 4 6 8 9 7 5 3 1

Manufactured in Hong Kong
on acid-free paper

# Preface

This atlas is intended for those interested in abnormal prenatal development in human beings and other mammals. This includes geneticists and developmental biologists, as well as those with a more applied interest, such as obstetricians, pediatricians, perinatologists, pediatric pathologists, toxicologists, and reproductive epidemiologists. Although abnormal human development caused by chromosome imbalance is usually studied only at the time of birth, the great majority of such imbalance leads to prenatal lethality, observable in humans as spontaneous abortions (also called miscarriages). The morphological spectrum characteristic of chromosome anomalies in these prenatal deaths is the subject of this atlas.

The material in the atlas was collected from 1974 to 1986 as part of a collaborative study of spontaneous abortion. The study began a few years after induced abortion was legalized in the state of New York. This event all but eliminated a major problem with previous studies of spontaneous abortion in this country, that is, the unknown number of illegal induced abortions that might be present in any collection of specimens. At that time two large chromosome surveys of spontaneous abortion had been completed, one in Paris by André and Joelle Boué, and the other in London by Michael Creasy and Eva Alberman. These studies confirmed David Carr's remarkable observation that a very large proportion of early miscarriages had chromosome abnormalities detectable under the light microscope. It was clear that anyone interested in the causes of chromosomal abnormalities—in particular the trisomy associated with Down syndrome, trisomy 21—would find ample material in the study of spontaneous abortions.

This led to the collaboration at Columbia Presbyterian Medical Center in New York City between Zena Stein and Mervyn Susser, epidemiologists interested in Down syndrome, and Dorothy Warburton, a human cytogeneticist with a longstanding interest in the epidemiology of spontaneous abortion. Also present at the outset was Jennie Kline, who began the study for her Ph.D. thesis project, and directed the project in its later years. The original study design consisted of the identification of all cases of spontaneous abortion in three Manhattan hospitals, a lengthy interview with all consenting women, and the collection of the abortion specimen and its culture for chromosome analysis whenever embryonic or fetal material could be identified. A set of control women drawn from deliveries after 28 weeks of gestation was also interviewed. A team of interviewers, data processors, and technologists was assembled to handle the 500 or so cases per year that were identified.

Julianne Byrne joined the group in 1977 as a research assistant enrolled in the Ph.D. program in epidemiology. At that time it had become clear that careful pathological examination and classification of the spontaneous abortion specimens were sources of information that were being overlooked. Intrigued by the potential in this largely undeveloped part of the study, and with the encouragement and support of William A. Blanc, head of

Developmental Pathology in Babies Hospital at Columbia Presbyterian Medical Center, she assumed the collection and analysis of the pathological data as her thesis project. The aim was to describe as fully as possible the gross morphology of the available abortion specimens, and to organize the material for analysis with respect to other variables in the study. A standard data collection form was developed, and fetal autopsy procedures were standardized. From 1977 to 1981 over 3,500 specimens were examined by Julianne Byrne with a succession of research assistants. Although full-scale fetal autopsies were not completed routinely after 1982, a classification scheme used by the cytogenetic technologists had been developed and basic information continued to be collected up to the end of the study.

Nina Canki, a pediatrician and clinical geneticist from Yugoslavia with an interest in embryonic and fetal pathology, joined Dorothy Warburton's laboratory as a Fullbright Scholar from September 1984 to September 1985. She intensively studied the new specimens, took many of the photographs that appear in this atlas, and added new insights to our observations both past and present. Nina Canki visited New York again in the winter of 1986 with the help of a grant from the March of Dimes Birth Defects Foundation to help organize the material of this atlas.

Our thanks are due to the many cytogenetic technologists who worked on the study, but especially to Chih-yu Yu, Marina Peters, Ming-Tsung Yu, and Raji Krishnamurthi whose long-term dedication to the project made it succeed. Marina Peters deserves special recognition because her interest and technical skill in examining the specimens alerted us to features we might otherwise have missed; she also took many of the photographs that appear in this atlas. We also thank Diane Baker, Debra Zillmer, Diana Andrews, and Phoebe Kussin who performed many of the autopsies; Dr. William A. Blanc and his staff and residents in the Division of Developmental Pathology where the material was analyzed; and Zena Stein, Mervyn Susser, Jennie

Kline, and Barbara Strobino, our principal collaborators in the study, for their friendship, guidance, and support. To Zena Stein we owe the initial realization that pathological examination should be explored in an epidemiological study. Dr. Phillip Ursell read much of the text and made many useful suggestions. Anita Lustenberger provided invaluable help in organizing the photographs, editing and analyzing the pathology data, and checking the references. Oxford University Press has also recently published *From Conception to Birth: Epidemiology of Prenatal Development*, 1990, by our collaborators Jennie Kline, Zena Stein, and Mervyn Susser. This text summarizes much of the epidemiological data from our spontaneous abortion study.

We hope that the specimens on these pages will intrigue as well as inform. Although molecular biology has provided such marvelous breakthroughs in the understanding of biological processes, it is humbling and thought provoking to realize how little we know about the course of events leading to the pathology illustrated in these pages. We do not understand how chromosome imbalance leads to abnormal and predominantly lethal outcomes, nor why the same chromosome change can demonstrate variable effects ranging from complete lack of an embryo to a full-term pregnancy. We also do not know by what signals genetic abnormalities compatible with development of a grossly normal placenta and embryo lead to premature labor and spontaneous termination of the pregnancy. Equally mysterious are the processes leading to numerical chromosome abnormalities via defects in cell division and gametogenesis. Our study and others have failed to find clear associations of chromosome abnormalities at conception with either environmental or genetic factors, with the notable exception of the association between trisomy and maternal age. Even here our understanding does not go beyond the epidemiological description of a phenomenon that has been well known for 50 years.

In most publications of pathological studies of spontaneous abortions, the few illustrations that accompany the text are black and white with limited detail. We present the sum of our many years of experience on the correlations between the chromosome constitution and the morphology of the aborted specimen in an atlas filled with as many color plates as permitted by our editors at Oxford. Our hope is for this atlas to find a home in the laboratories and offices of those interested in abnormal human development, and for it to help them interpret what they see, as well as encourage them to look.

Funding for this study was provided in part by grants ROI HD 08838, ROI HD 12207, ROI DA 02090, and ROI HD 15909 from the National Institutes of Health, and a grant from the March of Dimes Birth Defects Foundation.

*New York*                                                            D. W.
*Bethesda*                                                              J. B.
*Slajmerjeva, Yugoslavia*                                              N. C.

# Contents

# Chromosome Anomalies and
# Prenatal Development: An Atlas

# CHAPTER 1

# Background and Methods
# of this Study

Spontaneous abortions, or miscarriages, occur in 15–20% of all recognized human conceptions, that is those in which at least one missed menstrual period has occurred (Warburton, Fraser, 1964). Since these losses involve specimens that can be studied pathologically and genetically, the specimens have been widely used as a source of information about normal development and the causes of miscarriage.

Earlier embryonic losses are much less amenable to direct study. There is now good evidence, based on sensitive early pregnancy tests, that at least as high a proportion of conceptions are lost between implantation and the first missed menses (Wilcox et al., 1988). However, collection of embryonic tissues from these early losses would be very difficult, and no recent study has reported genetic or pathological research from this time period. The extent of even earlier human losses, between conception and implantation, can only be guessed at. The advent of in vitro fertilization as a medical procedure will undoubtedly open up some areas for observation, and reports of cytogenetic studies of very early conceptions and gametes are beginning to provide information on the rates of chromosome abnormalities at conception. (Angell et al., 1986; Martin et al., 1987; Martin, Rademaker, 1987; Brandriff et al., 1985; Wramsby et al., 1987; Pellestor, Selè, 1988).

Interest in early prenatal human loss has increased recently for several reasons. First, in developed countries, the modern family is usually small, planned, and often delayed until the parents are in their thirties. The loss of one or several planned conceptions therefore has a much larger impact on a couple trying to have children within a limited time period. Not realizing how common such early pregnancy losses are, they may search for an explanation of what they perceive to be a problem with themselves or their doctors. They are interested in tests such as a chromosome analysis that can shed light on the cause of their loss and its chance of recurrence. Doctors also are becoming more aware of the status of the embryo and fetus as they can examine it with ultrasound throughout pregnancy, and can sample fetal tissues at various stages for prenatal diagnosis of fetal conditions. Often "spontaneous" abortion is replaced by elective pregnancy termination after ultrasonographic diagnosis of an absent, dead, or moribund embryo or fetus, or one with serious congenital anomalies.

## Studies of Chromosome Abnormalities
## in Miscarriages

Quite soon after accurate human chromosome analysis became possible, chromosome anomalies in spontaneous abortion were described (Penrose, Delhanty, 1961). The work of David Carr (1967) in Canada, however, first indicated the very large fraction of human embryonic and fetal loss that could be attributed to aberrations in chromosome number and structure. This was followed by several large-scale epidemiologic, cytogenetic, and pathologic investigations, first in France by Joelle and Andre Boué (1973), then in Geneva (Kajii et al., 1973), Denmark (Lauritsen, 1976), London (Creasy et al., 1976), Canada (Poland et al., 1977), Japan (Takahara et al., 1977), Hawaii (Hassold et al., 1980) and New York City (Warburton, Stein et al., 1980).

All these studies provided a consistent picture of the extent and distribution of the various types of cytogenetic abnormalities. About 50% of first trimester spontaneous abortions have chromosome abnormalities; in studies such as ours that included later abortions, the proportion falls to about 40%. Abnormalities of number predominate, with *trisomy* (one extra normal chromosome) occurring in about 25% of all karyotyped early abortions. Next most frequent (about 7% each) are *monosomy X* (a missing sex chromosome) and *triploidy* (an entire extra chromosome set). *Tetraploidy* (two chromosome sets) and changes involving chromosome *rearrangements* also occur, but are much rarer (about 2% each). Almost no autosomal monosomies have been found among spontaneous abortions, and it is assumed that conceptions with this anomaly are lost before pregnancy is recognized. Chromosomal abnormalities are much more common in human conceptions than in other well-investigated mammals such as mice or rabbits (Maudlin, Fraser, 1978). The reasons for this are unknown, although it has been suggested that a high rate of early pregnancy loss may have provided a natural means of family size restriction—an advantage to a species with such a long and intensive rearing period (Warburton, 1987).

The large number of cases studied has also made it possible to examine associated factors such as parental age and recurrence risk, specifically with regard to the cytogenetic status of the spontaneous abortion. Increasing maternal age is associated with a roughly exponen-

tial increase in the rate of trisomic conceptions, and a decrease in the rate of conceptions with monosomy X in some settings. Most studies support a higher recurrence risk for spontaneous abortion in couples where a karyotyped abortion is chromosomally normal (Warburton, Strobino, 1987), and there is little increased recurrence risk for the same kind of chromosome anomaly in successive spontaneous abortions (Warburton et al., 1987; Morton et al., 1987). Although several studies specifically looked for associations between environmental factors and chromosomally abnormal conceptions, no consistent associations have been found except for the relationship between increased maternal age and trisomy (Kline, Stein, 1985).

In clinical practice the prognostic significance of the karyotype of the abortus is important, but cytogenetic studies on all miscarriages are currently impractical. It would thus be extremely useful if the morphological presentation of the specimen could be used to predict an abnormal karyotype, or, even better, a particular kind of abnormal karyotype. There have been numerous attempts to correlate specific chromosome anomalies with specific changes in morphology of the abortion specimen and some relationships have been demonstrated (Boué et al., 1976; Poland, Miller, 1973; Geisler, Kleinebrecht, 1978). Investigation of pathologic changes in the placenta has led to a recognition of some patterns specific to types of chromosome anomalies, such as triploidy with hydropic villi, or partial mole (Phillipe, 1973; Honoré et al., 1976; Jacobs et al., 1982). However, recent attempts to predict the karyotype from microscopic changes in the placental tissues have not shown this to be a very useful technique (Minguillon et al., 1989; Rehder et al., 1989).

From these observations and our own analysis of the New York study (Byrne et al., 1985) we can draw several important conclusions.

1. The phenotypic expression of a particular karyotypic abnormality may be extremely variable, ranging from conceptions expelled early in pregnancy with

only extraembryonic fetal tissues to conceptions surviving gestational life as newborns with congenital anomalies.

2. The pathological presentation cannot be used to precisely diagnose the presence or absence of a chromosome anomaly, nor the particular kind of anomaly present.

3. Nevertheless, there are striking differences among types of chromosome anomaly in the *distribution* of various kinds of pathological presentations. These may useful in defining the usual timing of developmental errors and causes of embryonic or fetal death.

Although there has been recent evidence that "imprinting" may lead to different phenotypes depending upon the parental source of additional or missing chromosomal regions, there is as yet no data to assess this source of variability among the karyotypic abnormalities presented here (Reik, 1989).

## Organization of the Atlas

This first chapter discusses the types of observations that will be presented, and compares these among karyotype groups using a series of histograms to depict the data. Subsequent chapters are arranged according to each type of chromosome abnormality in the order: monosomy X, triploidy, trisomy, and tetraploidy. Each chapter opens with a brief description of the entire series of specimens with that chromosome anomaly, with respect to the distribution of specimen type, gestational age, maternal age, chorionic villus type, and interactions between these characteristics. For specific anomalies additional points also need to be addressed, such as differences among trisomies for different chromosomes, and the distinctions between triploids with different sex chromosome complements. Comparisons among karyotype groups are addressed more completely in this introduction.

The bulk of each chapter consists of photographs of specimens, all of which come from our own collection.

Each specimen carries our identifying number, which is included for purposes of cross-referencing. The caption describes the notable features of the specimen, and also gives the fertilization age, when known, and the estimated developmental age. The captions for each picture are intended to aid in identifying the structures that are illustrated. In general, we have not included information about structures not visible in the photograph (e.g., internal anatomy, cord, or placenta). Since the photographs are those of specimens that happened to come into our collection, they do not necessarily provide a complete spectrum of the range of development nor of all the anomalies that can occur with any one karyotype. Among the trisomies, some of which are very rare, some karyotypes had few or no adequate photographs.

## Source of Cases

The material presented in this book was collected during a twelve-year (1974–1986) study of spontaneous abortions at three hospitals in New York City. Three parallel investigations were carried out whenever possible on each case of spontaneous abortion; an interview was conducted with the woman soon after the miscarriage; a cytogenetic analysis of the aborted tissues was attempted; and a gross pathologic examination of the aborted material was carried out. A team of interviewers identified women who came with a diagnosis of spontaneous abortion to one of the clinics or private doctors' offices at any of the three hospitals. Spontaneous abortion was defined as termination of pregnancy of a nonviable conceptus before 28 weeks of gestation. Products of conceptions were collected whenever possible and taken to the cytogenetics laboratory where cultures from embryonic or fetal tissues were established for karyotyping. Since an attempt was being made to examine and preserve actual embryos and fetuses, tissue for karyotyping was usually taken from chorionic villi or membranes when only a small embryo was present. The interviewers abstracted hospital charts on all cases, and conducted structured interviews covering: demographic characteristics; reproductive, family and medical history; and behaviors such as smoking, alcohol, and caffeine intake, drug use, and contraceptive use. Our population of women reflected the neighborhoods served by the three large teaching hospitals in upper Manhattan and was very diverse: about 23% were USA-born African Americans; 37% were Hispanic; 26% were USA-born white, non-Hispanic; and 14% were none of these. Socioeconomic status also varied widely; about one third of the women had family incomes below the federal poverty guidelines.

Over the 12 years of the study we collected specimens containing fetal material on 5,163 cases: of these, 3,300 were successfully karyotyped. Overall, approximately 40% of karyotyped specimens had an abnormal chromosome complement, and it is these specimens whose characteristics are illustrated in this book. In a few isolated instances we have supplemented this material with selected specimens from induced abortions following prenatal diagnosis of a chromosome abnormality; all photographs are from miscarriages unless otherwise specified.

**Table 1–1** Chromosome Complements of All Karyotyped Spontaneous Abortions

|  | Number | % of Total |
|---|---|---|
| Normal | 1,988 | 60.2 |
| Autosomal trisomy | 645 | 19.5 |
| Sex chromosome trisomy (all XXY) | 8 | 0.2 |
| Mosaic trisomy 47/46 | 60 | 1.8 |
| Double trisomy (including mosaics 48/47) | 35 | 1.1 |
| Monosomy X | 201 | 6.1 |
| Mosaic monosomy 45,X/46,XX | 15 | 0.5 |
| Triploidy total | 185 | 5.6 |
|     XXX     84 | | |
|     XXY     99 | | |
|     XYY      2 | | |
| Hypertriploidy (including mosaics 69/70) | 13 | 0.4 |
| Tetraploidy | 65 | 2.0 |
| Hypertetraploidy (including mosaics 94/93/92) | 13 | 0.4 |
| Balanced structural rearrangements | 11 | 0.3 |
| Unbalanced structural rearrangements | 41 | 1.2 |
| Others (double anomalies, etc.) | 20 | 0.6 |
| Total | 3,300 | |

## Cytogenetic Analysis

Tissue was cultured from embryonic or fetal tissue (i.e., from chorionic villi, fetal membranes, or parts of the embryo or fetus itself); most were karyotyped from extra-embryonic tissues. Karyotypes were prepared using trypsin-Giemsa banding in all cases. Ten mitoses were analyzed per specimen unless mosaicism was suggested by a single cell, in which case another 10 cells were analyzed. Mosaicism was diagnosed only if two similar nonmodal cells were found. In this atlas we have not included data on specimens with sex chromosome trisomy, mosaic karyotypes, structural rearrangements, or various kinds of double anomalies. The complete listing

of abnormal karyotypes in the 3,300 specimens successfully analyzed is given in Table 1–1.

## Photography

Photomicrographs for smaller specimens were made with a 35-mm camera attachment to a Wild M5 photomicroscope using Kodachrome 64 film and a fibreoptic light source. Larger specimens were photographed against a blue background using a Nikkormat camera attached to a ratcheted stand and fitted with a 50-mm lens and an adapter to achieve a 1:1 magnification. The photographs in this atlas represent examples from our collection that we feel are representative or that illustrate particular features; although they are not always of optimum quality, they do illustrate what can be observed in a routine examination of such specimens. All photography was completed under standard laboratory conditions by the primary examiner, either one of the authors, or a laboratory technician. No photographs were taken under studio lighting conditions.

## Morphological Study

We attempted to obtain all specimens unfixed because of the need to culture tissue for cytogenetic analysis; therefore all measurements were made and autopsies completed on unfixed tissue. For small specimens, examination usually occurred after immersion in Hank's balanced salt solution to prevent dehydration and to aid visualization. The dissecting microscope was used to view details of small specimens. In general, all fetuses longer than 50 mm were autopsied: however, some smaller fetuses and embryos were also autopsied. Morphological data was recorded on a standard form on all embryos, fetuses, and placentas (as in Byrne, 1983). Specific developmental anomalies were identified with the help of descriptions and photographs such as those in Nishimura and Okamoto (1976). Histological studies were not done routinely except in cases of special interest.

At the initial examination, each specimen was classified into one of a number of morphological classes depending upon the completeness of the specimen, the presence of fetal membranes or a cord, the presence or absence of an embryo or fetus, and the size of the embryo or fetus. For the analysis presented in this atlas many of these categories were condensed into fewer and larger groups depending on the degree of developmental organization achieved (Byrne et al., 1985). Table 1–2 shows this classification scheme. It begins with the least-organized specimens and proceeds to those that had the

**Table 1–2** Morphological Classes of Spontaneous Abortions

| Class | Morphology |
|---|---|
| 1 | Fragments of placenta only, or part of a ruptured sac without a cord |
| 2 | An intact empty sac without any visible embryo |
| 3 | A small disorganized embryo, 1–10 mm in length, usually attached directly to the amnion or chorion (GD-1 in Byrne et al., 1985) |
| 4 | A sac, ruptured or intact, containing a well-formed cord but without an embryo or fetus, or with only a fragment of embryonic tissue at the end of the cord (GD-2 in Byrne et al., 1985) |
| 5 | An embryo of 10–30 mm with or without visible malformations |
| 6 | A fetus, defined as being longer than 30 mm, with or without visible malformations |

greatest degree of development. All specimens were classified before cytogenetic analysis revealed the karyotype.

Specimens in class 1 were incomplete specimens, sometimes obtained after dilatation and curettage, and could have been derived from any of the other types of complete specimens. They are, however, more often found associated with chromosome anomalies compatible with only rudimentary embryonic development (Byrne et al., 1985), and are more likely to be derived from less-developed specimens such as classes 2 and 3 than from those with well-developed cords, embryos, or fetuses.

Figure 1–1 shows the distribution of morphological categories among specimens grouped by karyotypic abnormality. Because trisomy 16 was so much more frequent than other trisomies, itself as common as monosomy X or triploidy, this trisomy has been considered separately.

Among abortions with a normal karyotype, approximately 50% were fetuses: only about 10% had very rudimentary development (classes 2 or 3). On the other

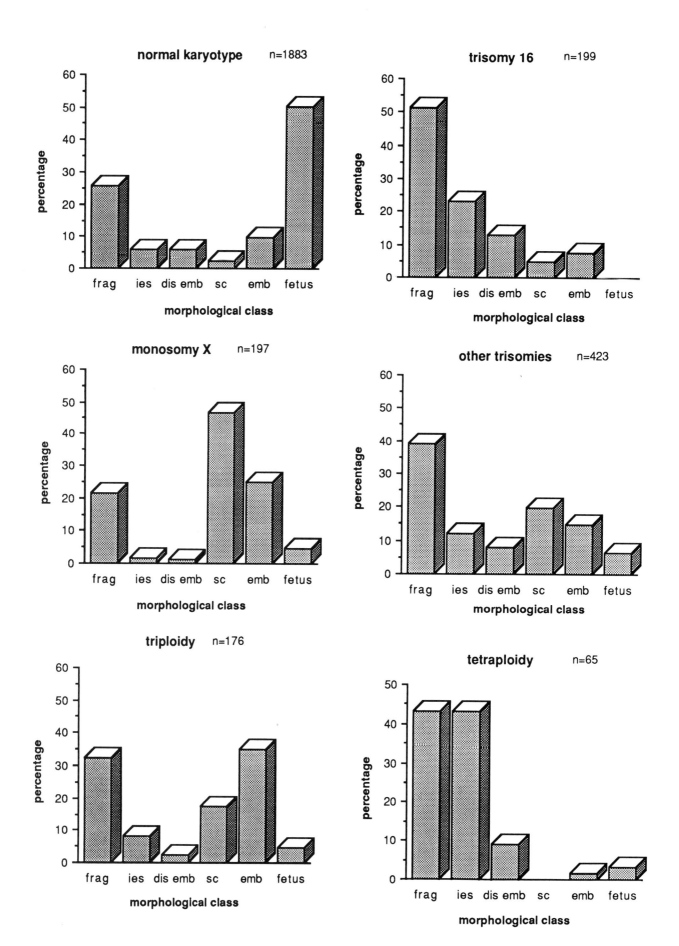

hand, among abortions with karyotypic abnormalities, fetuses comprised less than 10% of specimens. In the monosomy X group just a few complete specimens showed only very rudimentary development, with the predominating classes being those with a well-developed cord with or without an embryo or embryonic fragment. Among complete triploid specimens the most common presentation was as a well-developed embryo; however, more than 10% of specimens presented as intact empty sacs or rudimentary embryos. Trisomy 16 was never associated with development to the stage of a fetus, and presented most commonly as an intact empty sac or as a rudimentary embryo. The other trisomies were highly variable, as will be discussed in Chapter 4 on trisomies, some being compatible with fetal development and some achieving only rudimentary embryonic development. Tetraploid specimens were most commonly intact empty sacs.

## Estimation of Gestational and Developmental Age

Throughout the atlas we use *gestational age* as equivalent to the time elapsed since the last menstrual period (LMP); *fertilization age*, which is provided in the captions of the figures, was calculated by subtracting 14 days from the gestational age. In general, early spontaneous abortions are, of course, associated with less well-developed embryos and fetuses, although there

were numerous cases of "missed abortion" where a rudimentary or dead embryo was retained for many weeks after death. For this reason morphological status provides a better estimate of time of cessation of development than does gestation at abortion.

Figure 1–2 shows the distribution of gestational age at spontaneous abortion for the various karyotypic classes of specimen. For all types of specimens, except triploidy, there is a pronounced peak of gestational age at abortion around 10–12 weeks. This is most striking for monosomy X, where few specimens aborted earlier, and only a few cases survived into the second trimester. The gestation curve for triploidy is strikingly flat compared to that of the other karyotypes, but here again only a few cases survived beyond 18 weeks. Trisomies were more variable, although some cases (all trisomy 21 or 18) aborted later than 20 weeks.

Estimation of *developmental age* was attempted in all cases where there was an embryo or fetus. Accurate estimation of developmental age is necessary in order to distinguish between conditions that are normal at one stage of development and abnormal at another. For example, the presence of intestines in the umbilical cord is normal at nine weeks of development; after that the condition is classified as an omphalocele or umbilical hernia. Coloboma of the iris is normal up to 45 days, and the soft palate is not normally completely closed until about 10 weeks of development. Accurate estimation of developmental age poses many problems in cases of spontaneous abortion. Abnormal embryos may show asynchronous development, with some structures developing more slowly than others. Also, changes due to autolysis (maceration) and the trauma of delivery often distort structures such as the head and make it difficult to distinguish postmortem degeneration from abnormalities like neural tube defects. Although histological evaluation of such material may not often be useful, it is worth noting that even in severely autolyzed specimens the gross anatomy can be adequately assessed at autopsy.

Figure 1–1 Distribution (percent) of morphological classes for each major group of chromosome anomalies and for normal karyotypes. frag = fragments of placenta (group 1); ies = intact empty sac (group 2); dis emb = small disorganized embryo (group 3); sc = sac with cord but no embryo (group 4); emb = embryo 10–30 mm (group 5); fetus = fetus > 30 mm (group 6). Cases with unknown morphology are excluded.

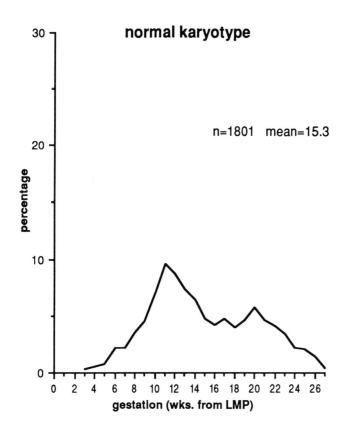

**normal karyotype**

n=1801    mean=15.3

percentage

gestation (wks. from LMP)

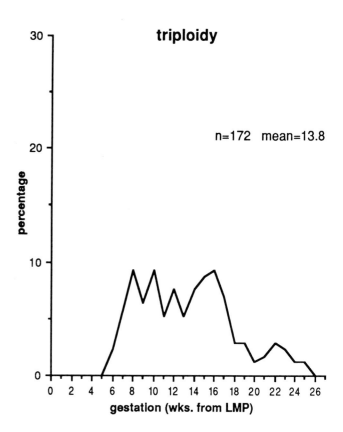

**triploidy**

n=172    mean=13.8

percentage

gestation (wks. from LMP)

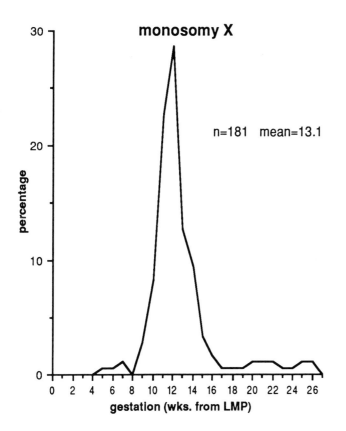

**monosomy X**

n=181    mean=13.1

percentage

gestation (wks. from LMP)

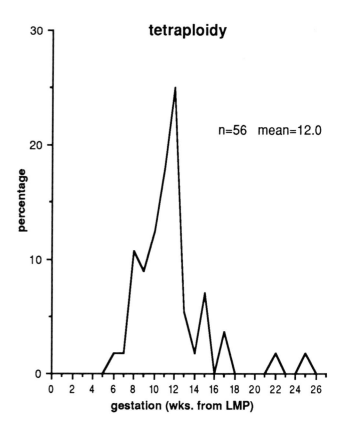

**tetraploidy**

n=56    mean=12.0

percentage

gestation (wks. from LMP)

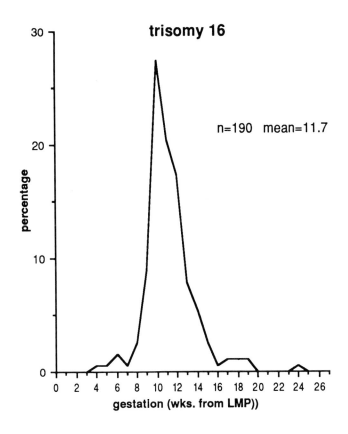

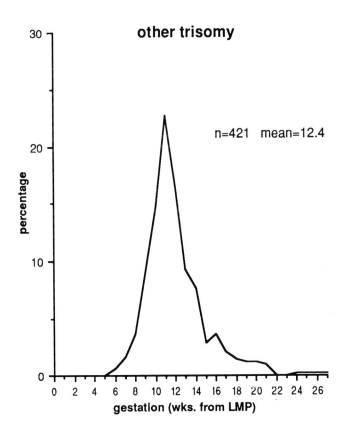

**Figure 1–2** Distribution (percent) of weeks of gestation for each major group of chromosome anomalies and for normal karyotypes. Cases with unknown gestation are excluded.

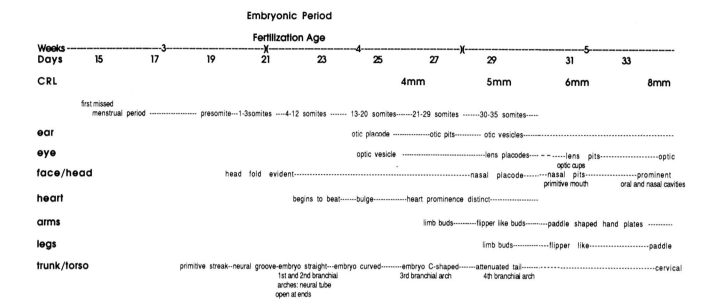

Figure 1–3 Major landmarks used in estimation of developmental age.

We used the developmental timetables provided by Moore (1988), O'Rahilly, Muller (1987), and Nishimura (1983) to determine the developmental stage that most closely matched the specimen at hand. When there were discrepancies between various features we decided to use the most advanced feature of the embryo, usually the crown-rump length (CRL), to date the specimen. The captions in the atlas point out numerous cases where development of one feature appeared retarded compared to others, for example: limb development may be retarded when compared with the development of the eye pigment. Figure 1–3 shows the major landmarks we used in estimating developmental age.

In general in these specimens, particularly the embryos, the retardation of development when compared with the fertilization age as estimated by LMP was striking. It was usually not possible to decide whether development proceeded at a reduced rate, or whether the embryo ceased development and died several weeks before expulsion; however, the degree of maceration of the specimen could sometimes help to make this distinction.

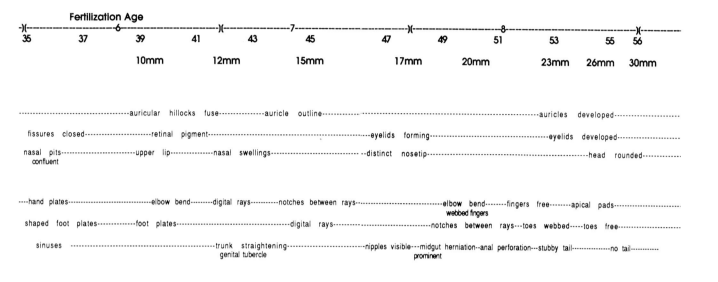

**Fertilization Age**

| 35 | 37 | 6 | 39 | 41 | 43 | 7 | 45 | 47 | 49 | 51 | 8 | 53 | 55 | 56 |

| 10mm | 12mm | 15mm | 17mm | 20mm | 23mm | 26mm | 30mm |

--------------------------------------------------auricular hillocks fuse----------------auricle outline-------------------------------------------------------------auricles developed----------------------

fissures closed-------------------------retinal pigment-------------------------------------------------------------eyelids forming-------------------------------------------eyelids developed--------------------

nasal pits---------------------------upper lip----------------nasal swellings-------------------------------distinct nosetip----------------------------------------------------head rounded------------
confluent

----hand plates---------------------------------elbow bend---------digital rays-----------notches between rays-----------------------------------elbow bend--------fingers free--------apical pads-------------------------
webbed fingers

shaped foot plates--------------foot plates---------------------------------------digital rays-------------------------------------notches between rays---toes webbed-----toes free---------------------

sinuses ------------------------------------------------------trunk straightening-------------------------nipples visible---midgut herniation--anal perforation---stubby tail---------------no tail----------
genital tubercle                                                                prominent

**Fetal Period**

**Fertilization Age**

| Weeks | 9 | 10 | 11 | 12 | 13 | 14 | 15 | 16 | 17 | 18 | 19 | 20 | 21 | 22 | 23 | 24 | 25 | 26 | 27 | 28 |
| CRL(mm) | 50 | 61 | | 87 | | 120 | | 140 | | 160 | | 190 | | 210 | | 230 | | 250 | | 270 |

**ear** ---------------------------------------------external ears stand out-------------------------------------------------

**eye** --------eyes closing--eyebrows---------------------------------------------------------------eyes opening-----------

**face** -- human profile-------------------------------------------------nostril opens------------------------------------
palate closing

**arms** ---early fingernails----------------------------------------------------------fingernails present------------------
dermatoglyphics

**legs** ---------------------------limbs well developed--------------------------------------------------------------toenails-----
early toenails

**trunk**---- ambiguous----well-defined neck --------------------mammary areolae---head and---skin red,-------lean body---------------------
external genitalia sexes distinguishable                                      body hair  wrinkled

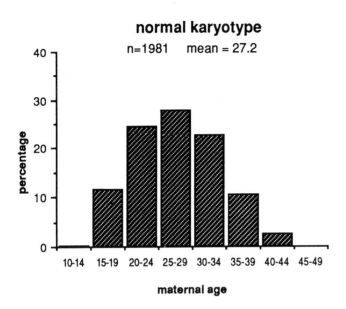

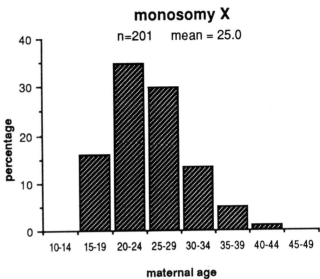

## Maternal Age

Maternal age was available for most specimens, and the distributions of maternal age for each karyotypic class are shown in Figure 1–4. We know the mean maternal age for chromosomally normal abortions is higher than that for livebirths in the same years (not shown in the figure). Triploid and tetraploid specimens showed a distribution similar to that of livebirths, indicating no effect of maternal age on the origin of these anomalies. For monosomy X the mean maternal age was about one year lower than those for triploidy and tetraploidy: for trisomy 16 it was about three years higher, and for other trisomies it was about five years higher. These maternal age associations are discussed in further detail in the chapters on the individual anomalies.

## Chorionic Villi

Examination of chorionic villi was introduced later in the study, and thus there are fewer cases with this information available. The chorionic villi were teased out from the chorion in Hank's solution and examined under the dissecting microscope. Villi were classified as normal, cystic, hypoplastic or clubbed, or occasionally as being derived from a true hydatidiform mole. Cystic villi were swollen, round, and lacking a core of connective tissues and blood vessels; hypoplastic villi were thin and lacked branching; clubbed villi had broad, cystic ends. The diagnosis of hydatidiform mole was made in specimens where no fetal membranes were present and all the villi were large and cystic. All villi were classified before knowledge of the karyotype.

In a specimen where more than one type of villus existed, which was not uncommon, the coding scheme allowed for only one choice. In this case, the villi were coded in the following order of preference: cystic, hypoplastic, clubbed, normal. The different kinds of chorionic villi are illustrated in Figure 1–5 (A–F). Other examples are found throughout the chapters on individual anomalies.

Figure 1–6 shows the relative frequencies of types of chorionic villi among specimens with a given karyotype. A significant proportion of chromosomally normal specimens were classified as having abnormal chorionic

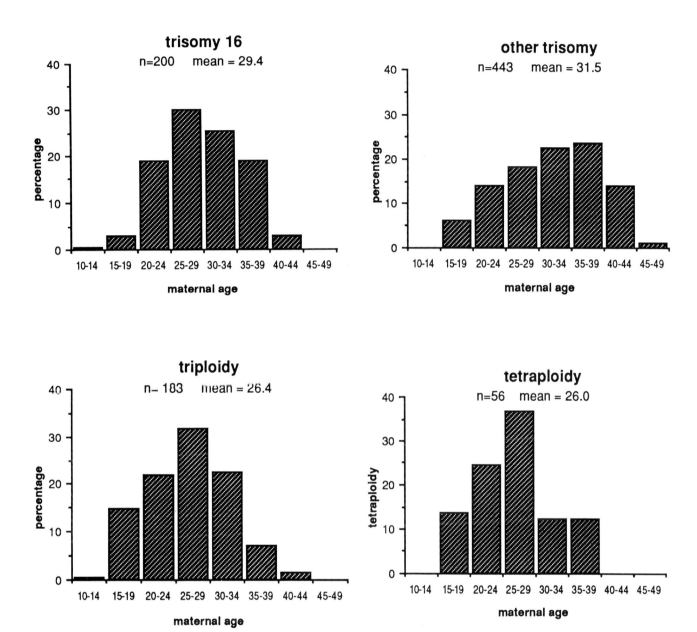

**Figure 1—4** Distribution (percent) of maternal ages for each major group of chromosome anomalies and for normal karyotypes. Cases with unknown maternal age are excluded.

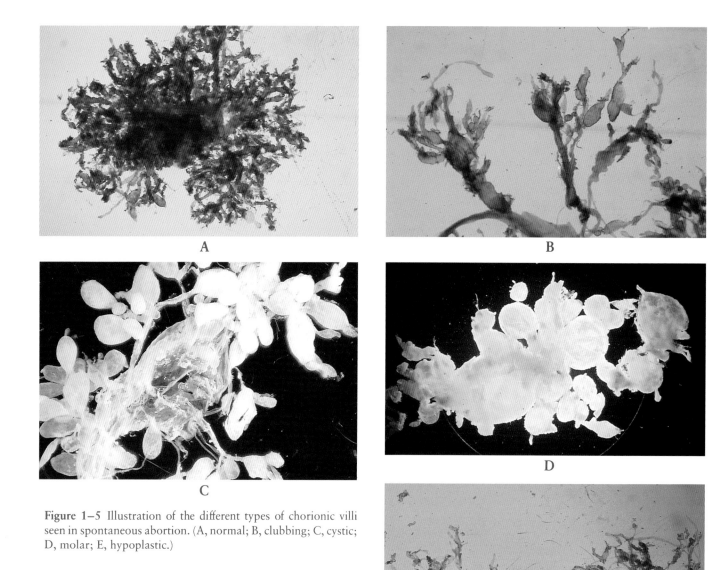

A

B

C

D

**Figure 1–5** Illustration of the different types of chorionic villi seen in spontaneous abortion. (A, normal; B, clubbing; C, cystic; D, molar; E, hypoplastic.)

E

villi. Hydatidiform mole, usually associated with a normal karyotype, was very unusual in our population. Among specimens with monosomy X, the predominant type of abnormality was hypoplastic. Among triploid specimens cystic villi were most common. Both these associations agree with observations by others (Philippe, 1973; Jacobs et al., 1982; Honoré et al., 1976). The trisomic specimens had a highly variable presentation of villi, with cystic villi being most common among specimens with trisomy 16.

**Figure 1–6** Distribution (percent) of types of chorionic villi for each major chromosome anomaly and for normal karyotypes. Cases with unknown villi type are excluded.

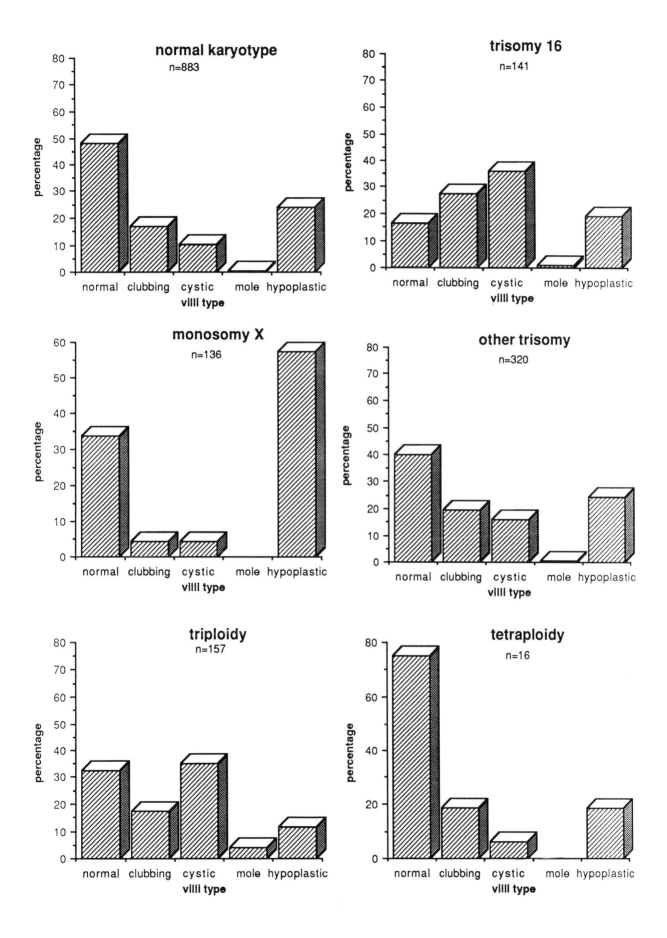

# CHAPTER 2

# Monosomy X

A total of 197 spontaneous abortions with only a single X chromosome (45,X) were classified by morphological type. The small number of other specimens with mosaicism for monosomy X or rearrangements of the X chromosome leading to partial X monosomy will not be considered in this summary.

## Distribution of Specimen Classes

Table 2–1 shows the distribution of specimen types among monosomy X cases. There were only 9 cases (6% of complete specimens) that presented as fetuses (over 30 mm in length). The smallest of these were 32- and 37-mm CRL respectively, and were morphologically sim-

**Table 2–1** Morphological Class Among Monosomy X Cases

|  | Number | % of Complete Specimens |
|---|---|---|
| Fragment | 42 | — |
| Intact empty sac | 3 | 1.9 |
| Small disorganized embryo (1–10 mm) | 2 | 1.3 |
| Sac with cord, embryo missing or fragment | 92 | 59.4 |
| Embryo or part of embryo (≤30 mm) | 49 | 31.6 |
| Fetus | 9 | 5.8 |
| Total cases examined | 197 | |

ilar to the embryos described below, without major malformations. In one fetus only portions of the limbs were received. All of the six larger complete fetuses, ranging from 69- to 220-mm CRL, had the characteristics previously described as typical of fetal monosomy X (Figs. 2–12 through 2–16): large cystic hygromata, lymphedema of the hands and feet, generalized edema, ascites and hydrothorax with hypoplastic lungs, coarctation of the aorta (in four cases), and single umbilical artery (in three cases). Other developmental anomalies such as horseshoe kidney (Fig. 2–15), persistent left cardinal vein (superior vena cava), ventricular septal defect (Fig. 2–15) and anomalous subclavian artery (Fig. 2–16) were each seen in a single case.

The external genitalia in these fetuses were those of a normal female. The internal genitalia also appeared to be similar in size and shape to those of normal female fetuses of the same developmental age. Histological examination of the ovaries in two cases did not reveal any marked departure from the expected number of follicles and connective tissue, although interpretation was hampered by severe autolysis. However, streak gonads (Fig. 2–21) were seen on gross examination in the largest fetus. This was one of apparently monozygotic twins with a single chorionic sac: the co-twin had a 46,XX karyotype and was normal in appearance.

The largest group of monosomy X specimens (59% of complete specimens), were classified as belonging to class 4, that is a chorionic and amniotic sac containing a well-defined umbilical cord 20–30mm in length, often dilated, with a fragment of apparently embryonic tissue at its end (Figs. 2–1 through 2–4). Only three out of 92 such specimens were received with intact sacs: the rest were ruptured. The tissue fragment appeared to be the remains of a severely autolysed embryo that had broken off. Sometimes the detached or fragmented embryo was still visible (Figs. 2–6 and 2–7). More often it was either lost when the sac ruptured or was resorbed into the amniotic fluid. Although this specimen type was found in the other karyotype groups as well, it was most common in monosomy X. It appears that the embryo with monosomy X tends to become very fragile, and is predisposed to rupture its abdominal wall and detach from the umbilical cord. The fragility might be due to a pathological state such as hydrops, or might occur secondary to embryonic death with subsequent maceration. The dilatations of the cord (Figs. 2–4 and 2–7), which are also often seen, may be part of the same process.

The second most common group of monosomy X specimens (32% of complete specimens) were small, usually macerated, embryos of 35–45 days developmental age, with gestational ages ranging from 70–150 days. Pronounced retrognathia and a reduced nasofrontal angle (Fig. 2–9) were often noted, and two embryos with encephalocele were observed (Fig. 2–7 and 2–10). The majority of these embryos, however, were apparently morphologically normal.

It is noteworthy that very few specimens with monosomy X showed only rudimentary development (empty sacs or very small embryos). Apparently the 45,X karyotype is usually capable of supporting fairly normal development for at least 5–6 weeks.

## Gestational Age at Abortion

The mean gestational age for all spontaneous abortions with monosomy X was 91.6 days. There is a pronounced mode at 10–13 weeks, with 60% of cases terminating at this time, and only 5% terminating earlier

(see Fig. 1–2). This lack of very early losses contrasts strikingly with the situation in triploidy, where there were almost equal numbers of spontaneous abortions at all weeks of gestation from 7–17 weeks. Although trisomic cases had a gestational distribution more similar to that in monosomy X, a higher proportion of cases (15%) terminated before 10 weeks.

## Maternal Age

The mean maternal age for monosomy X specimens was 24.5 years, about 1.5 years lower than that for livebirths in the same time period (a statistically significant difference). Only 20% of mothers were older than 30, as contrasted with 32% for triploid specimens, and 62% for trisomic specimens (Fig. 1–4). While there were no statistically significant differences in maternal age among specimens in different morphological categories, the mean maternal age for the nine specimens classified as fetuses was only 21.9 years.

## Chorionic Villi

In 57% of the cases, the gross morphology of the chorionic villi was described as hypoplastic, in 34% as normal, and in only 4% as cystic or clubbed (Table 2–2). The preponderance of cases with hypoplastic villi was unique to the monosomy X karyotype; the only other karyotype group with a substantial proportion of

Table 2–2 Distribution of Types of Chorionic Villi in Monosomy X

|                      | Number | % of Total |
|----------------------|--------|------------|
| Normal               | 46     | 33.8       |
| Cystic               | 6      | 4.4        |
| Hypoplastic          | 78     | 57.4       |
| Clubbed              | 6      | 4.4        |
| Total cases examined | 136    |            |

hypoplastic villi was the viable trisomies. The mono-somy X cases with hypoplastic villi did not differ in gestation, morphological specimen type, or maternal age from those with normal villi.


## Discussion

In livebirths with monosomy X, analysis of Xg blood groups showed that the retained X chromosome was maternal in about 75% of cases (Sanger et al., 1977). More recent techniques using DNA restriction fragment length polymorphisms (RFLPs) have confirmed that monosomy X typically involves loss of the father's X or Y chromosome (Hassold et al., 1988). The existence of a reduced average age (23.8 years versus 29.6 years) in cases with a paternal X, as compared to cases where the X chromosome is maternal, suggests the existence of a nondisjunctional mechanism that is more frequent among younger than among older women (Hassold et al., 1988). An overall inverse maternal age effect has been described in some studies of monosomy X in spontaneous abortions, including our own (Kajii, Ohama, 1979; Warburton, Kline et al., 1980).

Apart from an earlier paper that described a large portion of our specimens with monosomy X (Canki et al., 1988), there are four other series of spontaneous abortions where the relative frequencies of morphological types of spontaneous abortions with monosomy X can be estimated. Three of the four (Creasy et al., 1976; Lauritsen, 1976; Takahara et al., 1977) were similar to ours in that a large fraction of specimens consisted of a ruptured sac with a cord but only fragments of embryo. In the series of Boué et al. (1976), two thirds of specimens had a similar phenotype but the sac was described as usually intact. This probably merely

reflects a difference in the way the specimens were collected. It does, however, suggest that the missing embryonic parts must usually be resorbed into the amniotic fluid rather than simply being lost upon rupture of the sac.

The cystic hygromata, edema, coarctation of the aorta, and horseshoe kidney have all been described in many other studies of fetuses with monosomy X (e.g., Singh, Carr, 1966; Boué et al., 1976). The earlier spontaneously aborted embryos which are intact do not show cystic hygromata, which apparently develop after nine weeks. The suggestion of facial dysmorphism in these embryos, and the presence of neural tube defects in some, are not features reported in fetal Turner syndrome. It has been suggested that the embryonic and fetal edema characteristic of monosomy X may be due to hypoplasia of the lymphatic trunk (Putte, 1977) or to early hypoalbuminemia (Sheppard et al., 1986), and it has been proposed that other defects such as coarctation and horseshoe kidney can be secondary to a primary edema. However cystic hygromata and lymphedema cannot be considered pathognomic for Turner syndrome because they occur in fetuses with other chromosome anomalies as well as those with normal chromosomes (Chervenak et al., 1983; Byrne et al., 1984).

The relatively mild abnormalities in full-term infants with Turner syndrome, as opposed to the high lethality of embryonic monosomy X, have led to the suggestion that the surviving infants are all mosaics with a normal cell line present at least in early embryonic life (Hecht, Macfarlane, 1969; Boué, Boué, 1980; Canki et al., 1988). Mosaicism with an XX or XY cell line was found in only 7% of spontaneous abortions with monosomy X, in contrast to the 40% mosaicism seen in livebirths with features of Turner syndrome (Hook, Warburton, 1983).

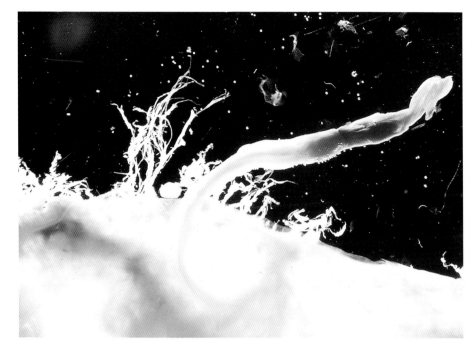

Figure 2–1 (4645) Umbilical cord attached to chorionic plate, showing necrotic fetal tissue fragment at the fetal end, received in a ruptured sac. Note the lack of branching in the hypoplastic chorionic villi extending up from beneath the cut edge of the specimen (Canki et al., 1988).

Fertilization age: 70 days

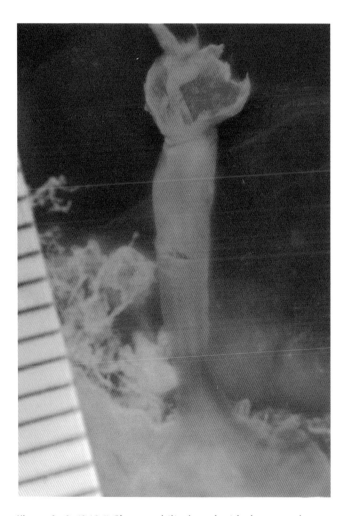

Figure 2–2 (2496) Short umbilical cord with three vessels containing fresh fetal blood. Parts of embryonic digestive system can be seen herniated into the cord at the ruptured distal end.

Fertilization age: 84 days

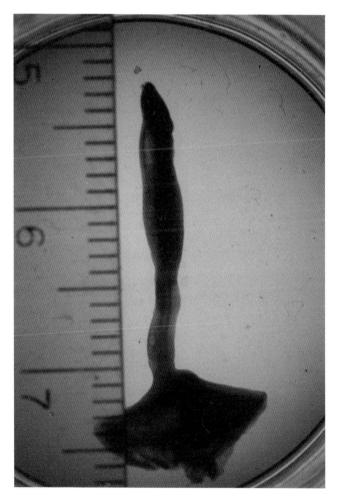

Figure 2–3 (2561) Autolysed umbilical cord with 2-mm piece of necrotic fetal tissue at upper end.

Fertilization age: 89 days

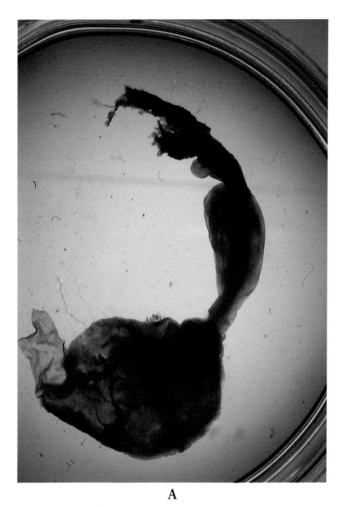

A

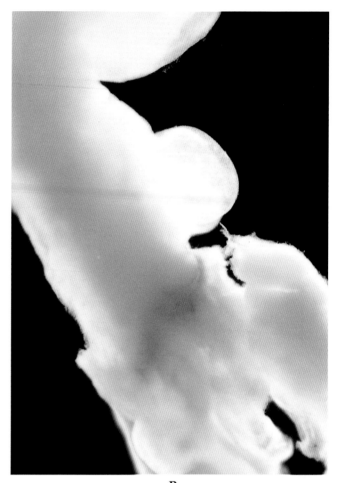

B

**Figure 2–4** (1798) (**A**) A 13-mm umbilical cord attached to the chorionic plate and membranes at the lower end with a necrotic brown 8-mm embryonic fragment at the distal end. (**B**) Closeup of free end showing part of cord and unidentifiable embryonic parts.

Fertilization age: 75 days

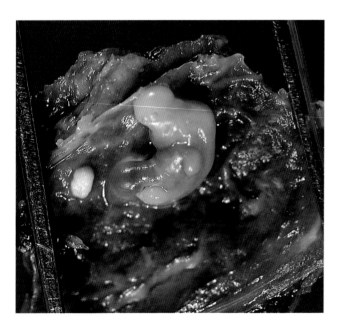

**Figure 2–5** (3312) A 13-mm CRL fixed autolysed embryo with pronounced cervical flexure, no retinal pigment, and flipperlike upper limb buds and identifiable lower limb buds. Note yolk sac remnant to left of short semitransparent cord. There is a discrepancy between the CRL and the developmental stage of eye and limbs.

Estimated developmental age: 41–43 days
Fertilization age: 90 days

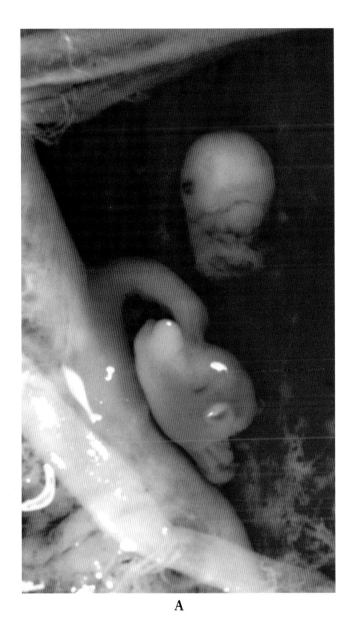

**A**

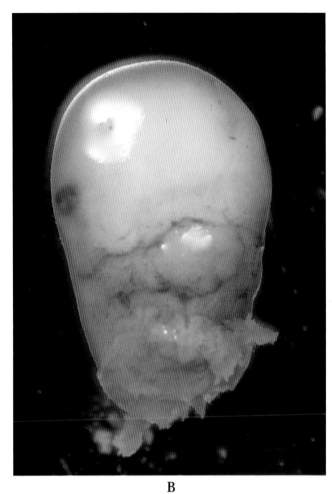

**B**

**Figure 2–6** (4479) (**A**) Two pieces of macerated embryo from intact chorionic sac. Retinal pigment is present, yet limb bud development is at an early stage. (**B**) Very autolysed head of specimen showing pigment in retina. Physiological coloboma is visible.

Estimated developmental age: 37–40 days
            Fertilization age: 65 days

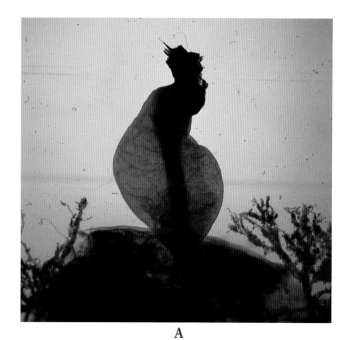

A

Figure 2–7 (4660) (A) Ruptured umbilical cord with lateral dilatations attached to amnion and chorionic plate. Two pieces of head and body of macerated embryo were found in the same ruptured sac. (B) Close-up of head showing parietal encephalocele, visible pigment in retina, abnormally shaped head or face, auricular hillocks (arrow). (C) Physiological cleft palate. Nares positioned normally relative to eyes and mouth (after fixation) (Canki et al., 1988).

Estimated developmental age: 37–41 days
　　　　Fertilization age: 68 days

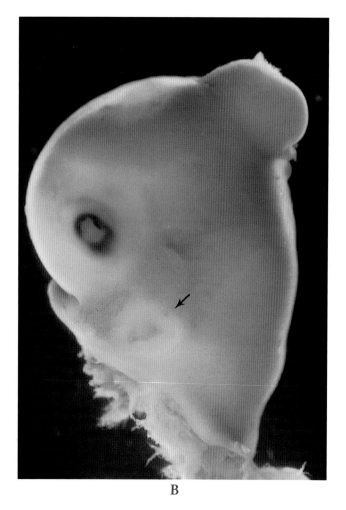

B

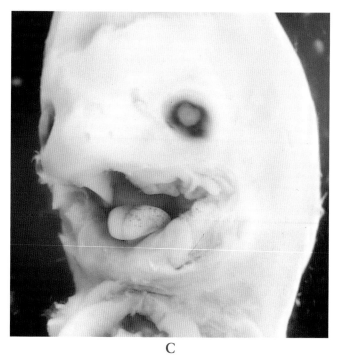

C

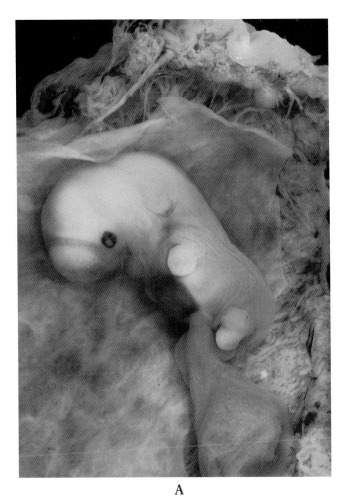

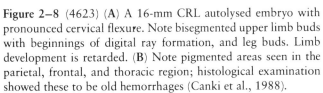

**A**

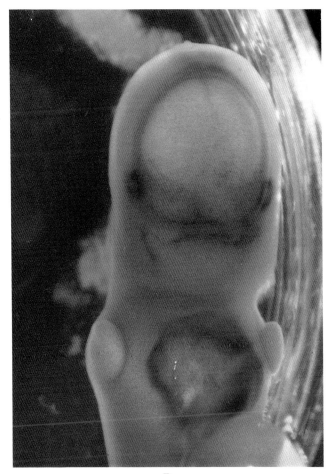

**B**

**Figure 2–8** (4623) (**A**) A 16-mm CRL autolysed embryo with pronounced cervical flexure. Note bisegmented upper limb buds with beginnings of digital ray formation, and leg buds. Limb development is retarded. (**B**) Note pigmented areas seen in the parietal, frontal, and thoracic region; histological examination showed these to be old hemorrhages (Canki et al., 1988).

Estimated developmental age: 44–48 days
        Fertilization age: 99 days

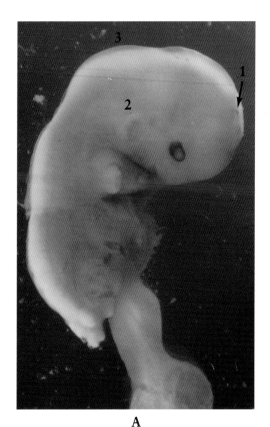

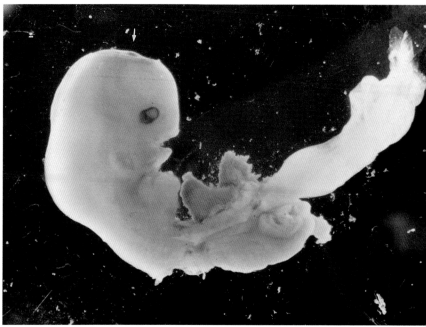

A

B

**Figure 2–9** (4565) (**A**) A 17-mm CRL embryo with dilated umbilical cord, distinct cervical flexure, pigmented flattened area at the top of skull (1), and retinal pigment. Auricular hillocks (2) are visible. Digital rays are present. There is a vesicular projection (nuchal bleb) in the region of the cervical flexure (3). (**B**) Lateral view after fixation and partial autopsy showing absence of nasofrontal angle and small lower jaw. Flattened area of subectodermal hemorrhage is present (arrow) (Canki et al., 1988).

Estimated developmental age: 44–46 days
Fertilization age: 71 days

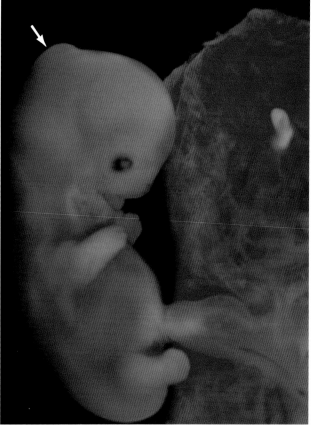

**Figure 2–10** (2833) A 23-mm embryo with parietal encephalocele (arrow), cleft palate (physiological?), and underdeveloped nasofrontal angle. The mandible is small. Digital rays are visible on upper limb, lower limb still paddle-shaped. Limb development is retarded for an embryo of this size. At least one well-preserved blood vessel is visible in cord (Canki et al., 1988).

Estimated developmental age: 52–53 days
Fertilization age: 68 days

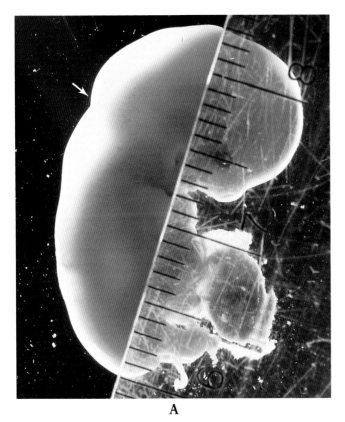

A

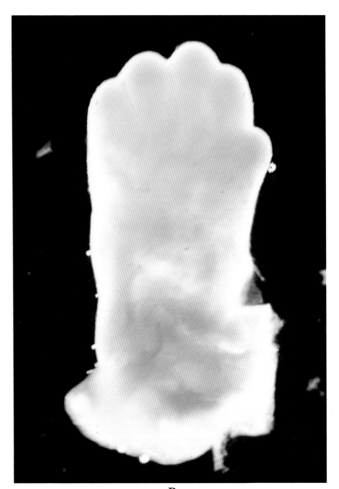

B

**Figure 2–11** (4628) (**A**) A 23-mm CRL embryo with nuchal bleb (arrow). Note abnormal head shape with reduced nasofrontal angle and small chin and physiological umbilical hernia. Eyelids are visible, and auricular hillocks are fused to form pinna. (**B**) On the hand plate note finger tubercles separated by interdigital notches. Digits are retarded in development for an embryo of this size. (**C**) Note nares and the cleft palate, which is normal for this stage of development (Canki et al., 1988).

Estimated developmental age: 52–53 days
        Fertilization age: 73 days

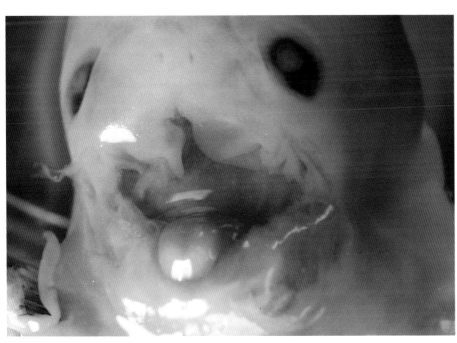

C

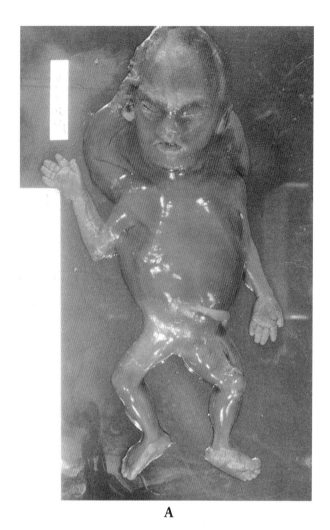
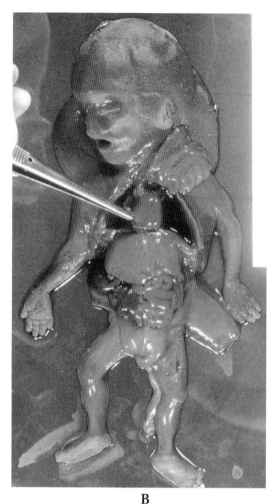

A

B

**Figure 2–12** (4541) (**A**) Severely autolysed 140-mm CRL fetus of 230 g with nuchal cystic hygromata and slight generalized edema. The cystic hygromata are asymmetric, larger on the right, and extended posteriorly and laterally to the shoulders following the insertion of the investing layer of cervical fascia. They consist of several noncommunicating chambers filled with brownish fluid. The hands and feet are slightly edematous. (**B**) Massive bilateral pleural effusion (about 4 ml on each side) with hypoplastic lungs and atrophic thymus. Note single (left) umbilical artery. (**C**) The thoracic duct (1) is apparently normally developed. The descending aorta (2) lies between it and the esophagus (3). (**D**) Dissection of heart and great vessels showing preductal coarctation of the aorta with a narrowing of the descending aorta superior to the ductus arteriosus: (1) ascending aorta, (2) arch of aorta, (3) preductal coarctation, (4) descending aorta, (5) pulmonic trunk, (6) right pulmonary artery, (7) ductus arteriosus, (8) vena cava superior, (9) left vagus nerve. The pulmonary arteries supplying the left lung (10) can be seen under the ductus. (**E**) Right hand, showing edema, and single flexion crease on second digit (Canki et al., 1988).

Estimated developmental age: 16 weeks
Fertilization age: 24 weeks

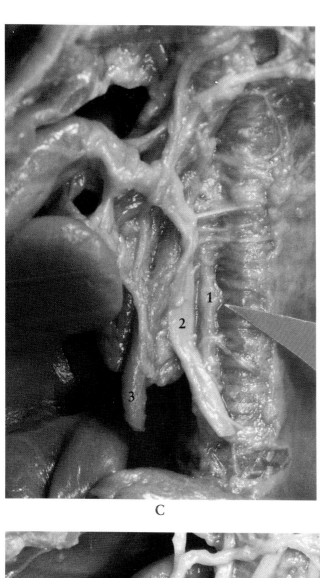

C

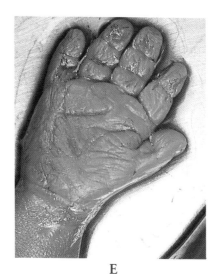

E

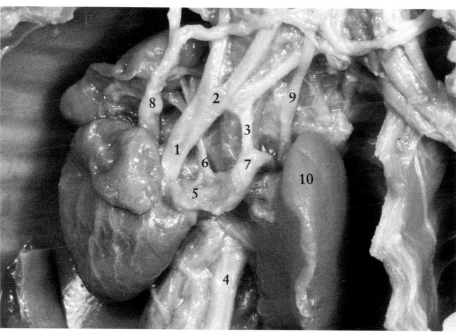

D

29

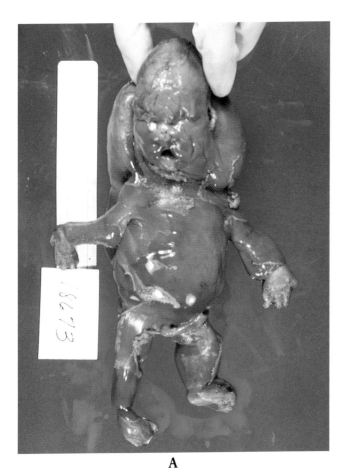

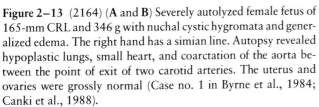

A

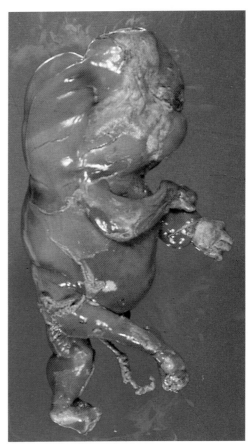

B

**Figure 2–13** (2164) (**A** and **B**) Severely autolyzed female fetus of 165-mm CRL and 346 g with nuchal cystic hygromata and generalized edema. The right hand has a simian line. Autopsy revealed hypoplastic lungs, small heart, and coarctation of the aorta between the point of exit of two carotid arteries. The uterus and ovaries were grossly normal (Case no. 1 in Byrne et al., 1984; Canki et al., 1988).

Estimated developmental age: 18 weeks
Fertilization age: 24 weeks

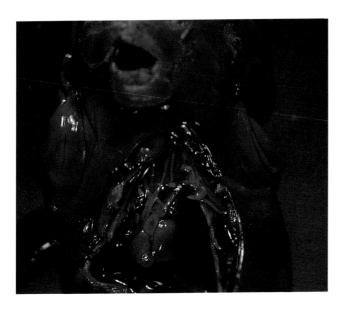

**Figure 2–14** (2751) Severely autolyzed edematous female fetus of 134-mm CRL and 275 g with cystic hygromata. Hygromata contain several noncommunicating cavities filled with brown fluid. The lungs and the heart are markedly small (0.9 and 0.5 g respectively) and there are pleural and pericardial effusions. There is tubular coarctation of the aorta, and partial malrotation of the gut (no right-sided attachment) (Case no. 4 in Byrne et al., 1984).

Estimated developmental age: 18 weeks
Fertilization age: 24 weeks

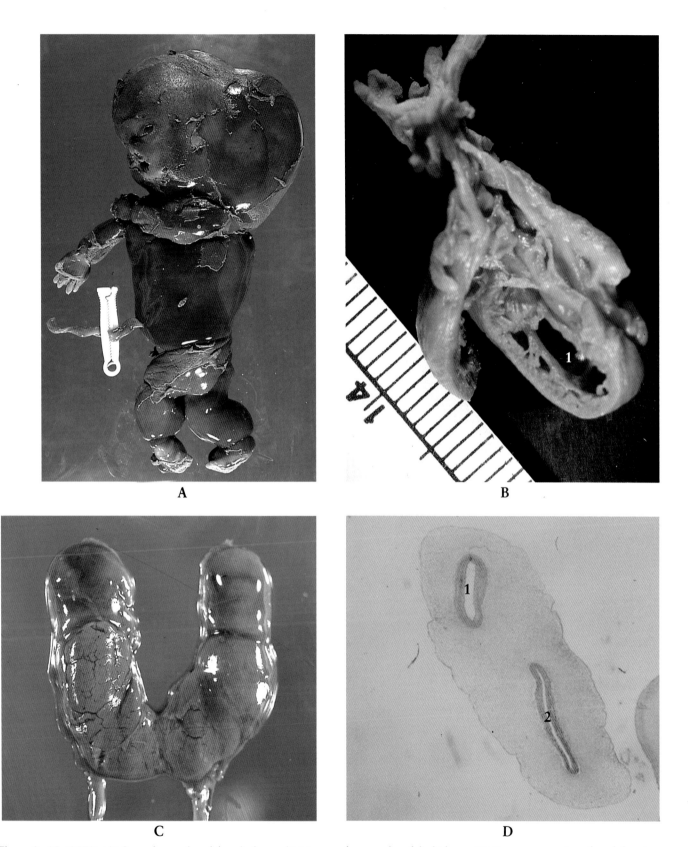

A

B

C

D

Figure 2–15 (2570) (A) Severely autolyzed female fetus of 195-mm CRL and 570 g. The bilateral cystic hygromata in nuchal region contained about 150 ml of fluid. Edema of upper and lower extremities is marked. On autolyzed skin, head and body hair are visible. (B) Right ventricular view. Muscular ventricular septal defect (1) of the "Swiss cheese" (multiple defect) type. (C) Posterior view of horseshoe kidney resulting from fusion of the lower poles of the kidneys. (D) Transverse section of cord showing single umbilical artery (1) and the umbilical vein (2) (Case no. 3 in Byrne et al., 1984; Canki et al., 1988.)

Estimated developmental age: 19–20 weeks
Fertilization age: 23 weeks

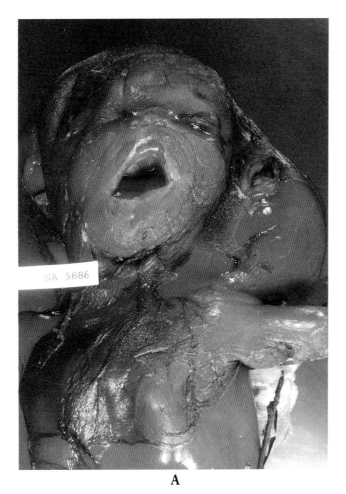

**A**

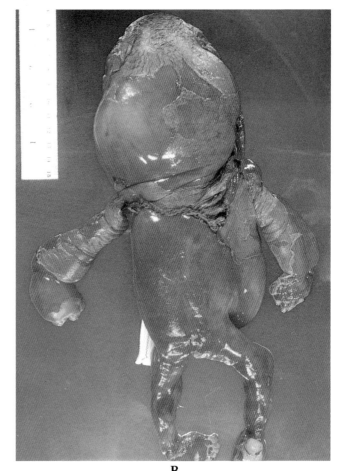

**B**

Figure 2–16 (4689) (**A, B,** and **C**) Macerated malformed female fetus of 220-mm CRL and 1340 g with karyotype 45,X, one of apparently monozygotic twins in a single chorion. There are huge bilateral cystic hygromata of the neck and lymphedema of most of the body. The facies is dysmorphic with small nose, flat nasal bridge, long upper lip, high palate, small posteriorly rotated mandible, dysplastic ears, and bilateral bridged simian crease. External genitalia appear to be normal female. (**D**) The right subclavian artery (1) has an abnormal origin, and is formed by the distal portion of the descending aorta (2) and the seventh intersegmental artery. (**E**) The umbilical cord has only two vessels, with a large left umbilical artery (1) and absent right umbilical artery, left internal iliac artery (2), uterus (3), urinary bladder (4) (Canki et al., 1988).

Estimated developmental age: 20 weeks
        Fertilization age: 22 weeks

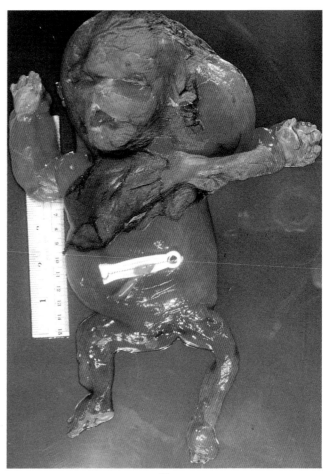

**C**

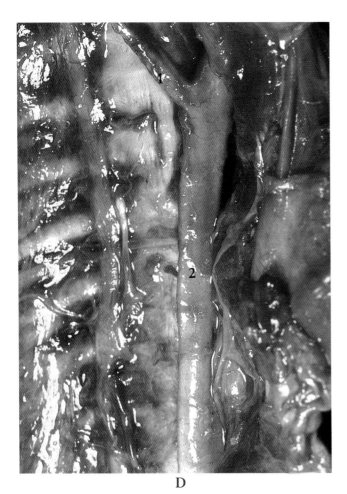

D

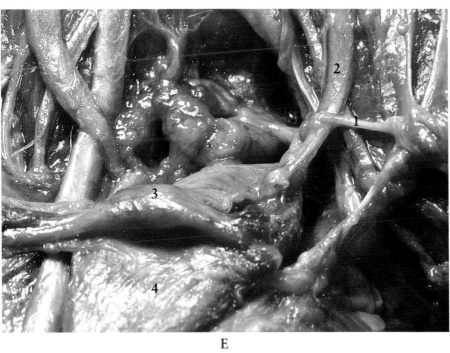

E

33

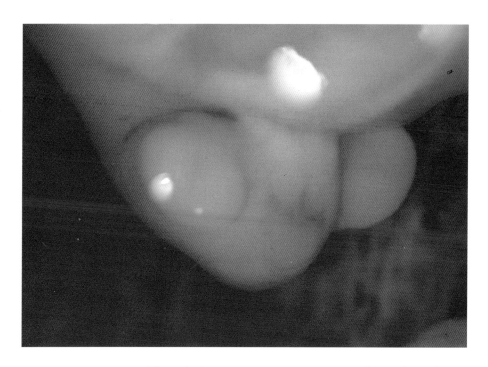

**Figure 2–17** (4479) (see Fig. 2–6) External genitalia at the undifferentiated stage.

Estimated developmental age: 37–40 days
Fertilization age: 78 days

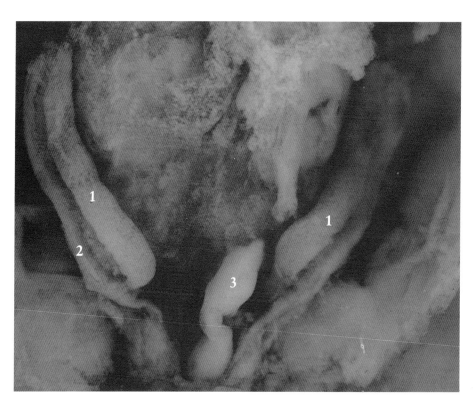

**Figure 2–18** (4446) Slightly more advanced stage of urogenital development: gonad (1), Mullerian duct (2), rectum (3).

Estimated developmental age: 51–53 days
Fertilization age: 70 days

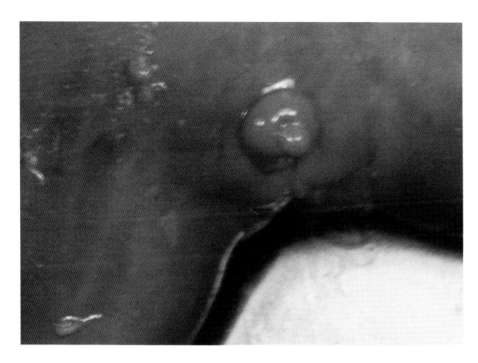

**Figure 2–19** (4541) (see Fig. 2–12). External genitalia show clitoris and labia majora.

Estimated developmental age: 16 weeks
Fertilization age: 24 weeks

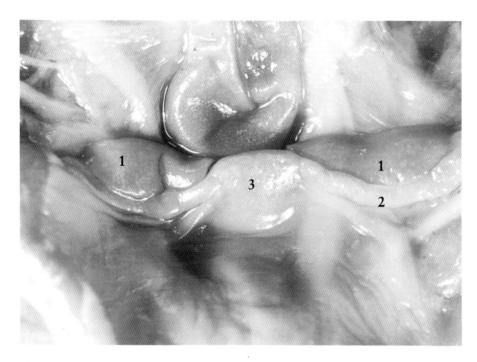

**Figure 2–20** (4541) (see Fig. 2–12) Ovaries (1), uterine tubes (2), and uterus (3) apparently of normal proportions. There is only the left umbilical artery.

Estimated developmental age: 16 weeks
Fertilization age: 24 weeks

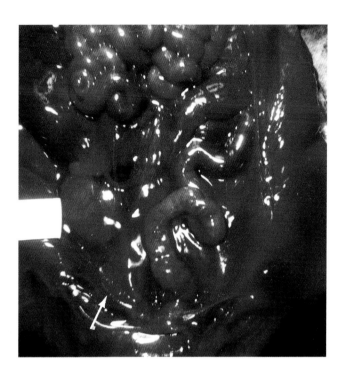

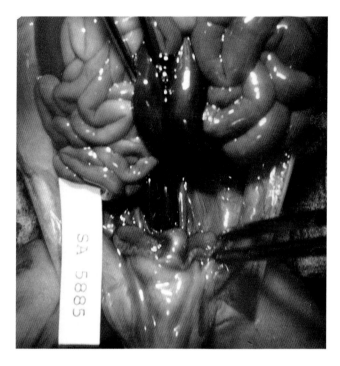

**Figure 2–21** (4689)B (see Fig. 2–16) Streak gonads (arrow) female twin with karyotype 45,X. A common mesentery and single right umbilical artery are also found.

Estimated developmental age: 20 weeks
                    Fertilization age: 22 weeks

**Figure 2–22** (4689) A (see Fig. 2–16). Normal ovaries from the co-twin with a normal female karyotype.

Estimated developmental age: 20 weeks
                    Fertilization age: 22 weeks

# CHAPTER 3

# Triploidy

A total of 176 triploid spontaneous abortion specimens were classified by morphological type. The sex chromosome distribution among all karyotyped specimens was XXX for 84 specimens, XXY for 99 specimens, and XYY for 2 specimens.

## Distribution of Specimen Classes

Table 3–1 shows the distribution of specimen classes among triploids with different sex chromosome complements. There were no significant differences between XXX and XXY triploids.

Only 6 XXX and 2 XXY triploids (7% of complete specimens) presented as fetuses over 30 mm in length. Those fetuses that were carefully examined had malformations, the most common being syndactyly, hydrocephaly, heart defects, hypoplastic kidneys and adrenals, and limb contractures (Figs. 3–21 through 3–25). These malformations are consistent with the features of the syndrome associated with triploidy in livebirths and fetuses diagnosed prenatally. One XXY fetus had normal male genitalia and gonads, while the other XXY fetus had apparently female external genitalia but normal male genitalia internally (Fig. 3–25), again consistent with reports of ambiguous genitalia in XXY triploid livebirths. One XXX fetus (Fig. 3–24) also had somewhat ambiguous external genitalia, no vagina or uterus, and small dysplastic ovaries.

The largest number of complete specimens (46% of XXX triploids and 60% of XXY triploids) consisted of

embryos less than 30 mm in length. These often appeared quite normal, (e.g., Figs. 3–12 and 3–13), but sometimes had visible malformations such as neural tube defects (Figs. 3–15, 3–16, and 3–20) or midline facial defects (Fig. 3–19). Brown spots indicating areas of old hemorrhage were common on the head and abdomen (Figs. 3–17 and 3–18). Although the fertilization ages of the pregnancies ranged from 4–21 weeks, the developmental age did not extend beyond eight weeks as estimated from CRL. In many cases severe autolysis indicated long retention of the embryo after death (Fig. 3–18). In other cases the embryos were not as severely autolyzed as the difference between developmental age and fertilization age would imply, suggesting that development had proceeded until shortly before expulsion, although at a greatly retarded rate (Fig. 3–13).

Only 18 complete specimens presented as intact empty sacs or very tiny disorganized embryos. Some of these were retained in utero for as long as 19 weeks after fertilization. Both of the XYY triploid specimens were intact empty sacs, in keeping with the hypothesis that such karyotypes are incompatible with significant embryonic development.

## Gestational Age at Abortion

The mean gestational age (weeks from LMP) for all triploid specimens was 97 days. There is a very broad

**Table 3–1** Morphological Class Among Triploids, by Sex Chromosome Complement

| | Fragments | Intact empty sac | Disorganized embryo | Sac with cord | Embryo | Fetus | All specimens |
|---|---|---|---|---|---|---|---|
| XXX triploids | 23 | 7 | 2 | 17 | 27 | 6 | 82 |
| % of all complete specimens | — | 11.9 | 3.4 | 28.8 | 45.8 | 10.2 | (59) |
| XXY triploids | 34 | 5 | 2 | 14 | 35 | 2 | 92 |
| % of all complete specimens | — | 8.6 | 3.4 | 24.1 | 60.3 | 3.4 | (58) |
| XYY triploids | 0 | 2 | 0 | 0 | 0 | 0 | 2 |
| % of all complete specimens | — | 100.0 | — | — | — | — | — |
| All triploids | 57 | 14 | 4 | 31 | 62 | 8 | 176 |
| % of all complete specimens | — | 11.8 | 3.4 | 26.1 | 52.1 | 6.7 | (119) |

and flat distribution of gestation (Fig. 1–2), with approximately equal numbers of specimens aborted at all weeks from 7 to 17. This is very different from the concentration of abortion at weeks 10 to 13 seen in all other karyotypes. There was no significant difference in gestational distribution for XXX and XXY triploids.

## Maternal Age

The maternal age for triploid spontaneous abortions of both XXX and XXY type in our sample was 26 years, which does not differ from the distribution of livebirths in the same time period. There was no difference among maternal age distributions for the various morphological categories of triploid specimens, and thus no suggestion that maternal age contributed to differences in developmental stage achieved before spontaneous abortion.

## Chorionic Villi

Chorionic villi were described as grossly cystic 38% of the time; 51% of the time they were described as normal or clubbed, and 11% of the time as hypoplastic. There was no apparent association of cystic villi with specimen type (Table 3–2) or with maternal age. Cystic villi were, however, identified more often in specimens of longer gestation: the mean gestational age for specimens with cystic villi was 105 days, while for specimens with normal villi it was 82 days. This suggests that the cystic villi develop or increase in number over the time a nonviable pregnancy continues.

Many previous studies have described the association of the triploid karyotype with cystic villi accompanied by a gestational sac (i.e., the so-called partial mole) (Philippe et al., 1980). Jacobs et al. (1982) showed that this was characteristic of but not restricted to triploids with two paternal chromosome sets. In our data, XXY

**Table 3–2** Types of Chorionic Villi by Specimen Type, Among Triploids

| | % of specimens classified as | | | | Number of specimens |
|---|---|---|---|---|---|
| | normal | cystic | hypoplastic | clubbed | |
| Fragment | 34.8 | 41.3 | 8.7 | 15.2 | 46 |
| Intact empty sac | 42.9 | 50.0 | 0.0 | 7.1 | 14 |
| Disorganized embryo | 33.3 | 33.3 | 0.0 | 33.3 | 3 |
| Sac with cord | 23.3 | 36.7 | 16.7 | 23.3 | 30 |
| Embryo | 32.7 | 32.7 | 15.4 | 19.2 | 52 |
| Fetus | 40.0 | 40.0 | 0.0 | 20.0 | 5 |
| Total examined | 32.7 | 38.0 | 11.3 | 18.0 | 150 |

triploids had cystic villi somewhat more often (46%) than did XXX triploids (33%), which is consistent with the fact that XXY triploids will have two paternal sets more often than XXX triploids. Although cystic villi are often found in triploid specimens, they cannot be considered diagnostic of triploidy: the same proportion of specimens with trisomy 16 were classified as having cystic villi on gross examination, and cystic villi were found in all karyotype groups. Of all specimens with cystic villi in our series, only 21% were triploid (compared to 7% of all specimens).

## Discussion

Although analysis of chromosomal polymorphisms of the parents and triploid conception can determine which parent has contributed two chromosome sets, we did not perform these studies for the majority of our cases. In two other series (Jacobs, Hassold 1980; Hunt et al., 1983; Uchida, Freeman, 1985), 77% and 62% of triploids respectively were shown to have two paternal chromosome sets, most often due to the fertilization of one oocyte by two sperm. Since approximately one-half of all sperm are X-bearing, and one-half are Y-bearing, one would expect dispermy to result in a ratio of 1 XXX triploid: 2 XXY triploids: 1 XYY triploid. Nevertheless,

the XYY sex chromosome complement is extremely rare, comprising only about 1% of all triploids in every study of spontaneous abortion. This suggests that such specimens are capable of very limited development, so that embryonic death usually occurs before recognized pregnancy. Triploids with two maternal chromosome sets can result from complete nondisjunction (retention of polar body) at either maternal meiosis I or II. In these situations equal proportions of XXX and XXY sex chromosome complements would be expected. The proportion of XXY to XXX triploids varies significantly among populations (Warburton, Stein et al., 1980). Our New York series has a relatively high proportion of XXX triploids; this may indicate that a much larger proportion of cases are due to diploid oocytes.

Our data are consistent with other reports of smaller series of triploid spontaneous abortions, although the proportion of specimens which are embryos of 10–30 mm is higher in our series than in those of Boué et al. (1976) or Creasy (1976). Boué states that developmental arrest is most common at 4–6 weeks, whereas more than half of our complete embryos had a CRL consistent with development to 6–8 weeks. However, this may not represent a real difference because estimates of CRL in the early weeks have been revised since the Boué study (Moore, 1988). Boué et al. (1976) also noted that neural tube defects and midline defects such as cyclocephaly were the chief malformations seen in embryos. Harris et al. (1981) described the most common features in a series of 40 triploid embryos to be facial dysplasia, subectodermal hemorrhage, cystic villi, and retarded limb development. We also found, in many of our embryos (Figs. 3–14, 3–15, and 3–18), that the developmental stage of the digits was earlier than that indicated by CRL or by the presence of retinal pigment. This phenomenon of asynchronous growth may not be restricted to embryos with triploidy: the same situation was found in embryos with monosomy and trisomy.

Since fetuses with triploidy can survive until the time of prenatal diagnosis by amniocentesis, several studies have considered the ultrasonographic features of tri-

ploidy. Retarded intra-uterine growth, relative microcephaly, and shortening of long bones has been reported (Lockwood et al., 1987b) and the condition is often accompanied by either cystic villi that can be seen ultrasonographically or complications of pregnancy such as preeclampsia, vaginal bleeding, or polyhydramnios (Graham et al., 1989). The physical findings of fetuses and livebirths with triploidy have been well described (Schinzel, 1984). They commonly include syndactyly, dysplastic kidneys, brain malformations, growth retardation, contractures of the joints, and ambiguities of the genitalia. Less frequent are neural tube defects, ocular defects, congenital heart defects, and omphalocele.

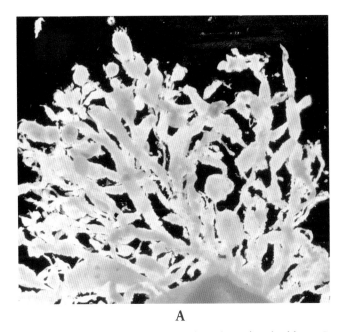

A

B

**Figure 3–1** (4727) (**A**) Normal villi with profuse budding. (**B**) Different region of same specimen: mostly hypoplastic pattern with occasional cystic villi.

Fertilization age: unknown
    Karyotype: 69,XXY

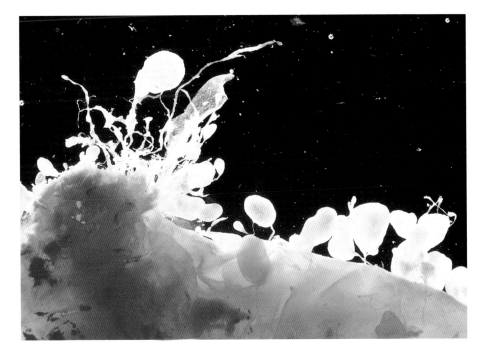

**Figure 3–2** (4726) Cystic villi with areas of hypoplasia.

Fertilization age: 19 weeks
    Karyotype: 69,XXX

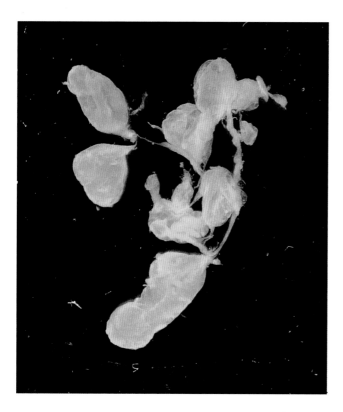

**Figure 3–3** (2606) Very large cystic villi, up to 3 mm in diameter.

Fertilization age: 12 weeks
    Karyotype: 69,XXY

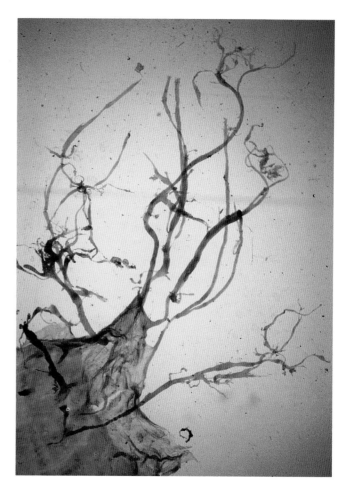

**Figure 3–4** (4654) Uniformly hypoplastic villi, long and thin with very little branching or budding.

Fertilization age: 20 weeks
    Karyotype: 69,XXY

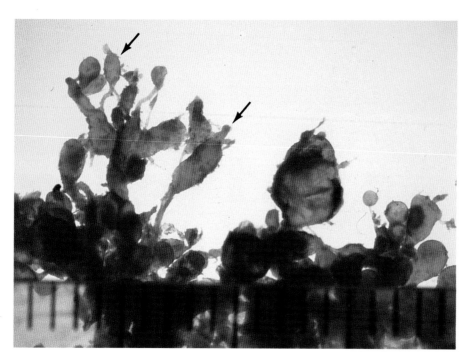

**Figure 3–5** (4669) Mixed pattern of cystic and clubbed (arrows) villi.

Fertilization age: 13 weeks
    Karyotype: 69,XXX

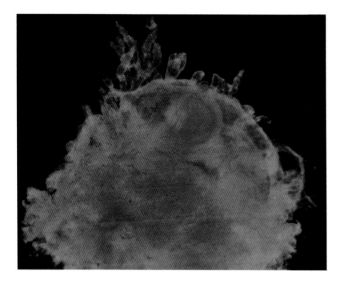

**Figure 3–6** (3514) Intact sac, 5 mm in diameter, covered with villi, with embryo and cord inside (not clearly seen in this picture).

Fertilization age: 37 days
Karyotype: 69,XXY

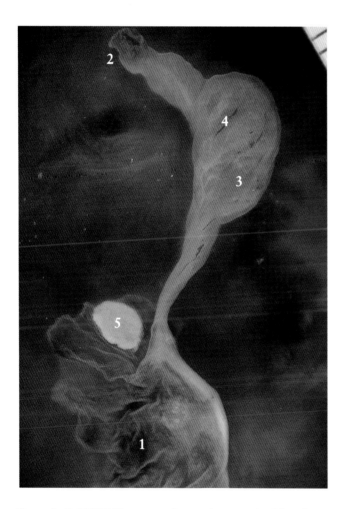

**Figure 3–7** (2502) Fragment of an embryo received in a large ruptured sac with extensive subchorionic hemorrhage (1). Villi were cystic. The 2-mm embryonic fragment (2) is at the end of a large dilated cord (3) 20 mm long and 8 mm at its greatest diameter. Note blood vessels in cord (4) and calcified yolk sac remnant (5).

Fertilization age: 10 weeks
Karyotype: 69,XXY

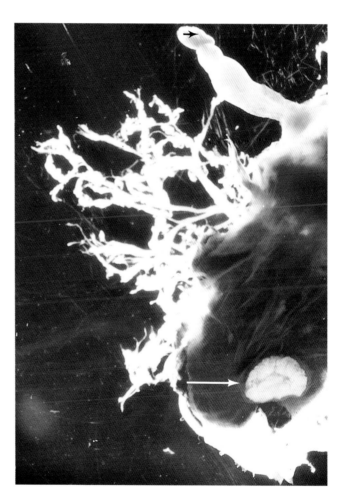

**Figure 3–8** (4591) Ruptured sac with embryonic fragment (small arrow) at the end of a macerated cord. Note hypoplastic villi and calcified yolk sac remnant (large arrow).

Fertilization age: 12 weeks
Karyotype: 69,XXY

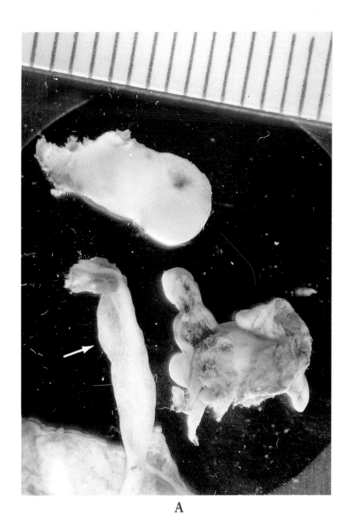

**A**

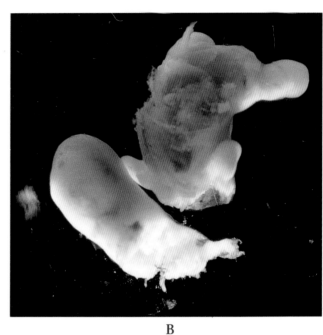

**B**

**Figure 3–9** (2559) (**A** and **B**) Embryo in two fragments, detached from cord (arrow) and quite autolyzed (13-mm total CRL). Upper and lower limbs are well developed but without digital rays. Eye pigment is present. (**C**) Cystic villi from same specimen.

Estimated developmental age: 41–44 days
Fertilization age: 119 days
Karyotype: 69,XXY

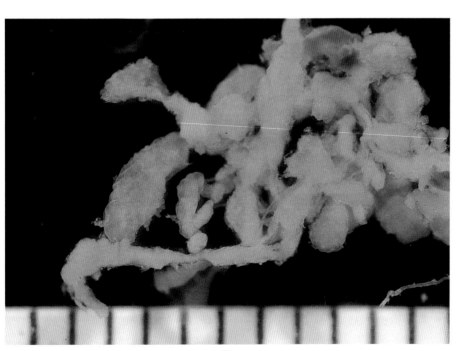

**C**

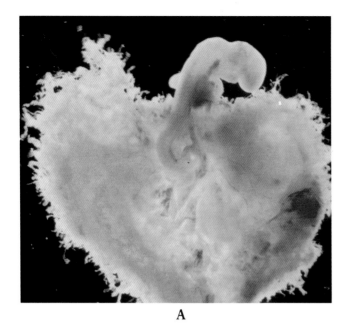

A

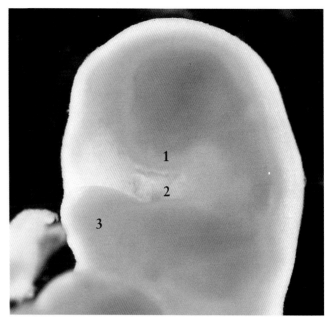

C

**Figure 3-10** (4549) A 9-mm CRL well-preserved embryo. (**A**) Opened sac showing embryo. (**B**) upper limb visible (1), heart prominence (2), cervical flexure just beginning (3) and eye without pigment (arrow). (**C**) Close-up of the face showing frontonasal elevation (1), stomodeum (2), and mandibular prominence (3).

Estimated developmental age: 33–36 days
Fertilization age: 43 days
Karyotype: 69,XXX

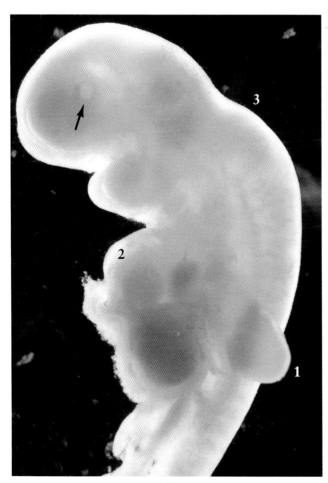

B

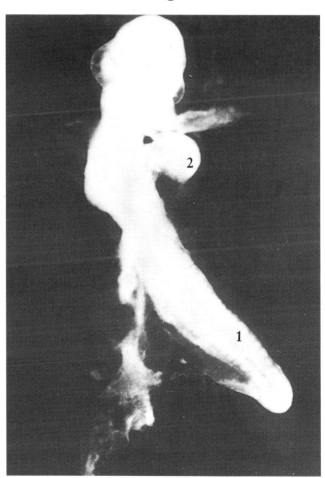

**Figure 3-11** (1436) A 4-mm CRL embryo received in an intact sac 10 mm in diameter. The embryo is well preserved with 13–20 somites (1), and heart prominence (2). No limb buds have developed at this stage.

Estimated developmental age: 24–25 days
Fertilization age: 39 days
Karyotype: 69,XXX

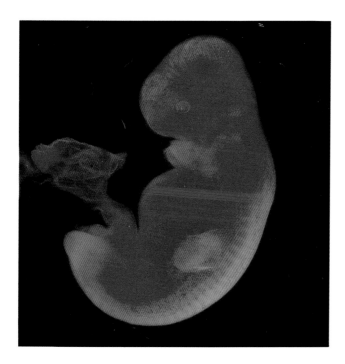

**Figure 3–12** (3463) A 10-mm CRL well-preserved embryo, with 25–30 somites, apparently normal in appearance. Upper limb buds clearly visible; lower limb buds just protruding beyond curvature of tail. Lack of pigment in eye suggests retarded development of this organ.

Estimated developmental age: 37–40 days
Fertilization age: 40 days
Karyotype: 69,XXY

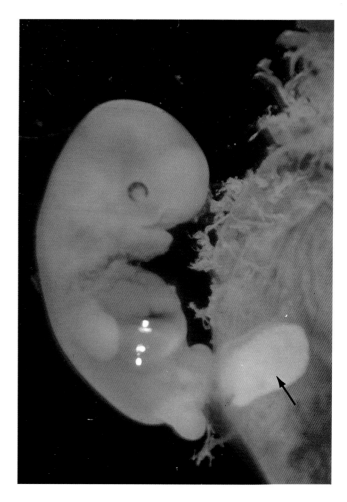

**Figure 3–13** (2391) A 13-mm CRL, slightly macerated embryo received in an intact sac with hypoplastic villi. Note 5-mm yolk-sac (arrow) attached to the amnion, and the pigmented eye. There was an hemorrhagic area on the back of the head not seen in this picture. Physiological coloboma is present.

Estimated developmental age: 41–43 days
Fertilization age: 108 days
Karyotype: 69,XXY

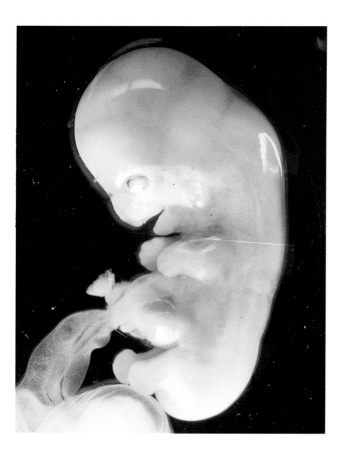

**Figure 3–14** (4498) A 22-mm CRL embryo, apparently normal, with a physiological umbilical hernia and three vessels in the cord. Reduced naso-frontal angle; poorly developed digits indicate retarded limb development.

Estimated developmental age: 49–51 days
Fertilization age: unknown
Karyotype: 69,XXX

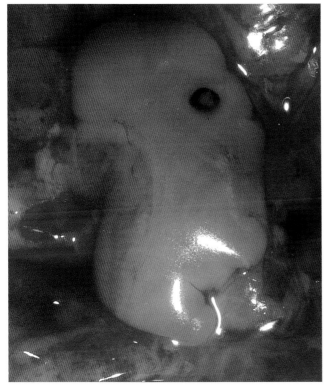

A

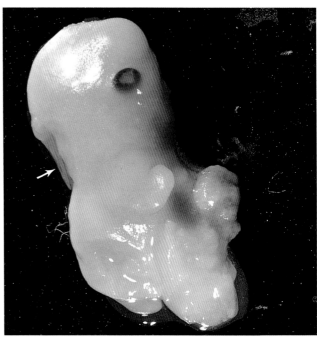

B

**Figure 3–15** (2894) (**A** and **B**) A 12-mm CRL embryo attached to the chorionic plate by a short body stalk. A lesion in the neck and spinal region is interpreted as a neural tube defect (arrow). Due to the retroflexion of the head and the peculiar appearance of the face, the NTD is characterized as iniencephaly. No finger or toe rays are seen on the limb buds, but the eye is pigmented and the optic fissure is closed. (Specimen no. 8 in Byrne and Warburton, 1986; specimen no. 23 in Table 5 in Byrne et al., 1985.)

Estimated developmental age: 42 days
Fertilization age: 71 days
Karyotype: 69,XXY

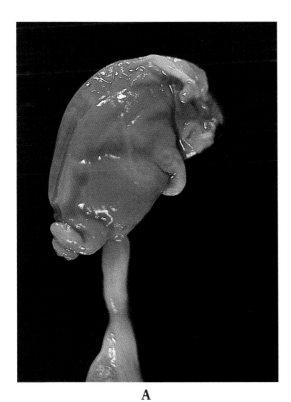

A

B

**Figure 3–16** (1163) (**A** and **B**) A 15-mm CRL very macerated embryo. The umbilical cord measures 20 mm with a 5 mm dilation. Embryo appears somewhat compressed laterally. The eyes appear to be on top of the head, the cranial vault is missing and the spine is open all the way to the sacrum. This is interpreted as anencephaly and spina bifida. (Specimen no. 24 (Table 5) in Byrne et al., 1985; no. 7 in Byrne and Warburton, 1986.)

Estimated developmental age: 44–46 days
Fertilization age: 125 days
Karyotype: 69,XXX

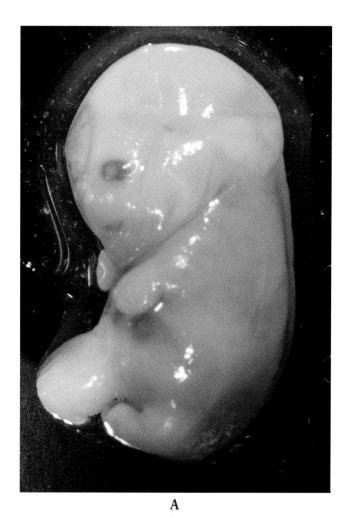

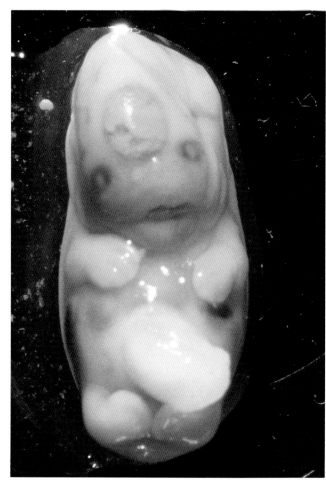

A                                                                  B

**Figure 3–17** (1239) (**A** and **B**) A 16-mm CRL embryo received in an intact sac. The embryo is severely autolyzed, and has a dark brown sharply circumscribed area above and between the eyes. This and several other circular brown areas on the body have been identified as areas of old hemorrhage on histological section. Digital rays are beginning to be apparent on the hands but not on the feet, which is retarded for an embryo of this size.

Estimated developmental age: 44–46 days
                Fertilization age: 126 days
                        Karyotype: 69,XXY

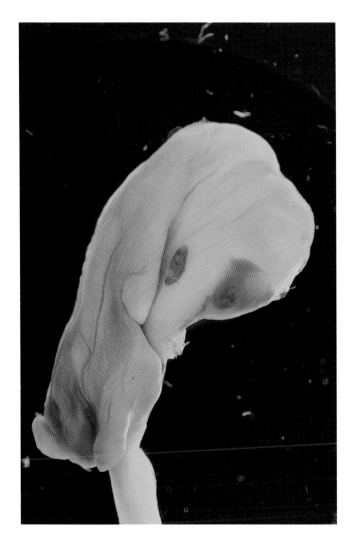

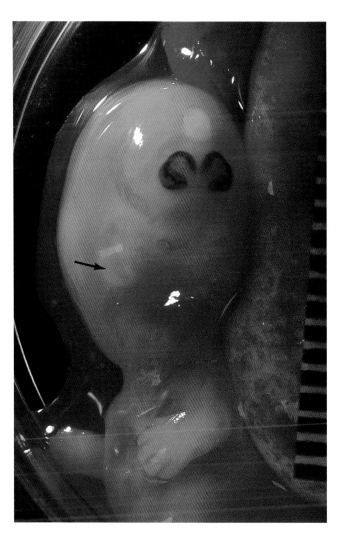

**Figure 3–18** (2750) A 15-mm CRL, very macerated embryo attached by cord to chorionic plate. The villi were cystic. Embryo is shrivelled but no focal malformation could be seen. There is a hemorrhagic area in the middle of the forehead, and another behind the lower limb.

Estimated developmental age: 44–46 days
Fertilization age: 96 days
Karyotype: 69,XXY

**Figure 3–19** (3467) A 20-mm CRL embryo with eyes very closely set together, each eye with coloboma. Auricular hillocks visible (arrow). Circular white area above the eyes may be a proboscis.

Estimated developmental age: 49–51 days
Fertilization age: 29 days (sic)
Karyotype: 69,XXY

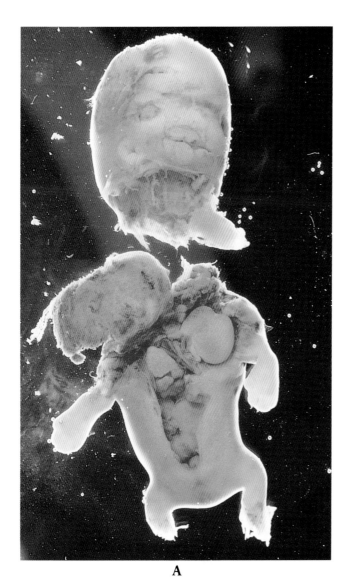

A

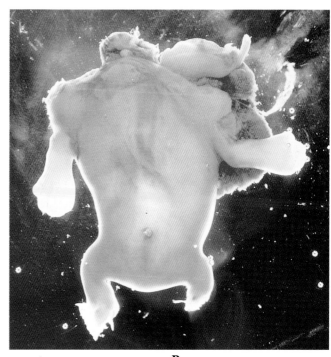

B

**Figure 3–20** (4635) (**A** and **B**) Severely autolyzed, fragmented embryo, with lumbar neural tube defect, apparently a meningocele. (**C**) Anterior view of pelvis, showing ambiguous external genitalia.

Estimated developmental age: 8 weeks
                Fertilization age: 12 weeks
                    Karyotype: 69,XXY

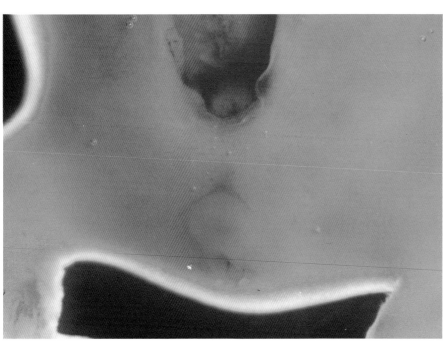

C

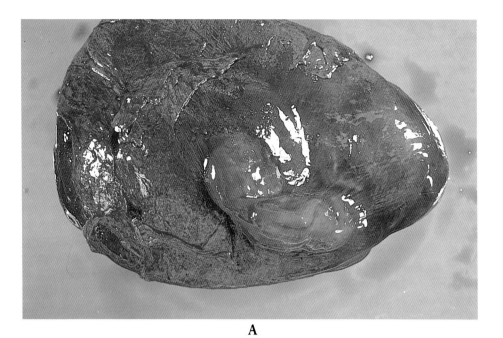

A

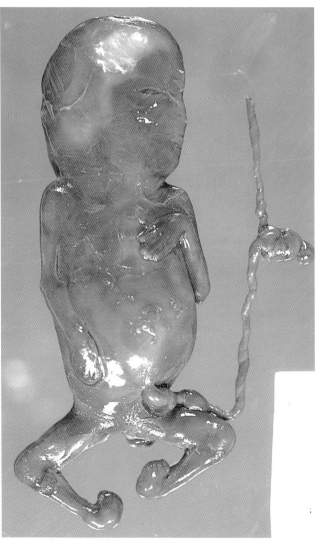

B

**Figure 3–21** (2482) (**A** and **B**) Very autolyzed and compressed 86-mm CRL fetus, with bilateral talipes and joint contractures (weight 27g). Received in a hemorrhagic placenta with intact membranes and long, thin cord; note false knot. Villi were cystic.

Estimated developmental age: 12 weeks
Fertilization age: 20 weeks
Karyotype: 69,XXX

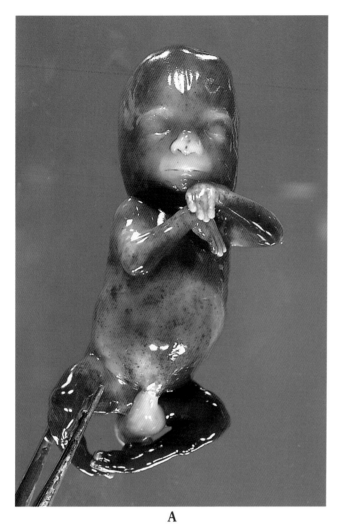

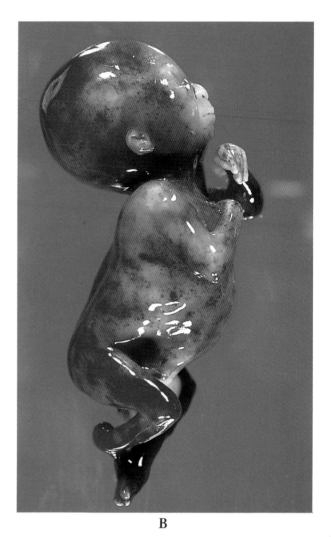

A

B

**Figure 3–22** (3596) (**A** and **B**) Well-preserved male fetus, weight 126 g, 117-mm CRL, slightly edematous. Head and face are nor-mal, chin is small. Both feet are clubbed and there are contractures of the upper limbs. There is a membranous ventricular septal defect. Adrenals are small with petechiae on the surface. Gonads are those of a normal male. (**C**) Edematous placenta, 130 × 100 × 20 mm. Cystic villi (arrow) up to 5 mm in diameter. Cord, 360 × 6 mm, is long and thin.

Estimated developmental age: 14 weeks
Fertilization age: 14 weeks
Karyotype: 69,XXY

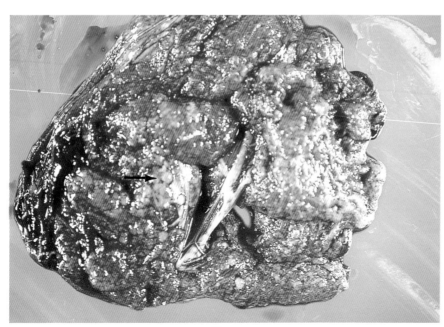

C

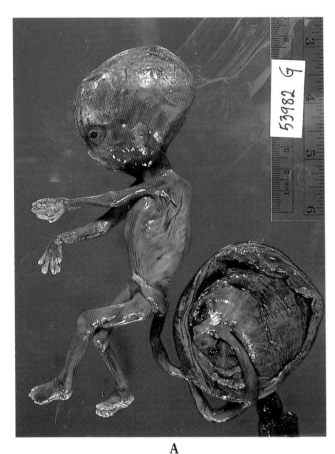

A

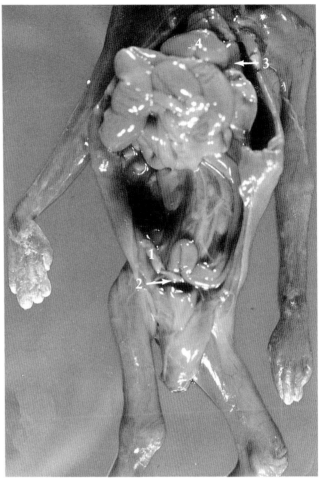

B

**Figure 3–23** (3343) (**A**) Fetus is attached to the small placenta by a long cord that contained only two vessels. The severely auto-lyzed fetus has hydrocephaly, and normal female external geni-talia. Weight 76 g and 124-mm CRL. Syndactyly of digits 2+3 on the right hand only; left hand is normal. Nose and chin are small, eyes are widespaced and open. (**B**) Dissection. Contents of ab-domen are reflected upwards and cover thorax. Note normal female genitalia, right ovary (1) and uterus (2). Lungs are small (3) without fluid in the pleural spaces. The heart is large (4), with a massive right atrium and a dilated coronary sinus. Persistent left superior vena cava. Right umbilical artery missing.

Estimated developmental age: 14 weeks
Fertilization age: 22 weeks
Karyotype: 69,XXX

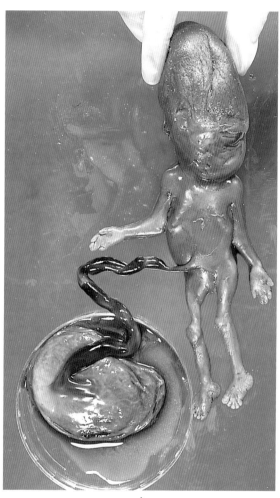

A

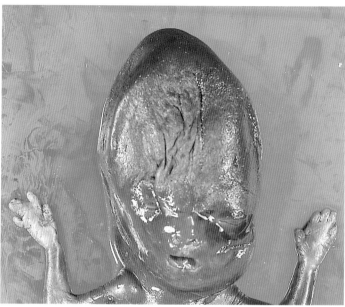

B

**Figure 3–24** (1447) (**A**) A 135-mm CRL fetus with small (70 × 55 × 6 mm) quite autolyzed placenta. Cord is very long and thin (185 × 6 mm) with only two vessels. Normal chorionic villi. Ambiguous external genitalia, appearing more female than male. (**B**) Large, apparently hydrocephalic, head. (**C, D**, and **E**) Hands and feet edematous, in contrast to an almost emaciated appearance of the rest of the body. Syndactyly of both hands and feet; digits 2+3+4 on both hands; digits 2+3+4+5 on the feet at least partly fused. (**F**) Internally, the genitalia are again ambiguous. Lungs (1) are hypoplastic; heart (2) is large with membranous ventricular septal defect. Both kidney (3) and adrenals (4) are small. No vagina or uterus; gonads seem to be represented by two masses of friable tissue (5). Left umbilical artery is missing.

Estimated developmental age: 13 weeks
Fertilization age: 21 weeks
Karyotype: 69,XXX

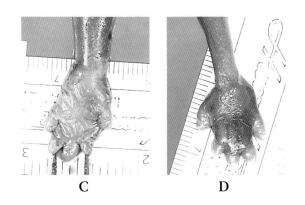

C D

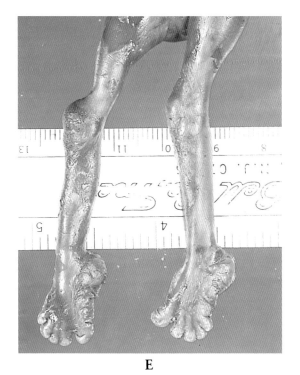

E

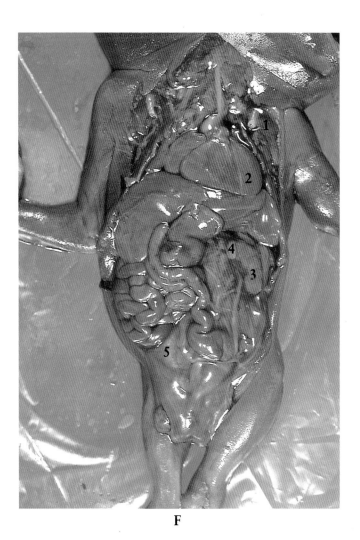

F

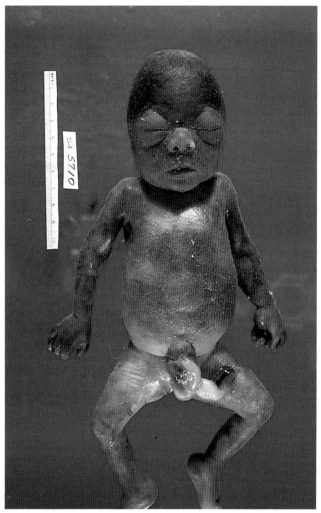

A

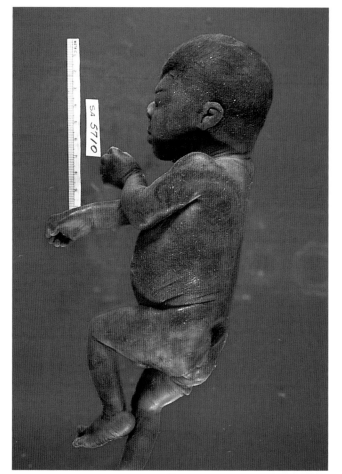

B

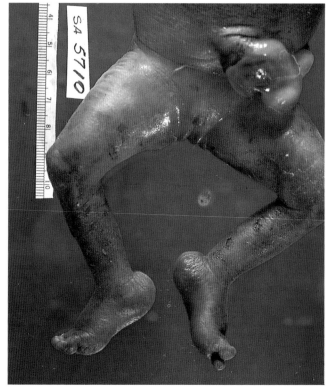

C

**Figure 3–25** (2813) The placenta of this well-preserved, malformed fetus had several unusual features: circummargination and circumvallation with a 25-mm rim of extra-chorial placenta, a large (154 × 190 × 10 mm) chorionic plate, and large trophoblastic cysts. A long cord, 40 × 8 mm, had three vessels. (**A** and **B**) Fetus is 190-mm CRL, 285-mm crown-heel length. External genitalia appear to be female but internal examination shows normal male testes. Face is remarkable for a depressed nasal bridge, anteverted nostrils, small mouth, periorbital edema, and midline frontal bossing. (**C**) Umbilicus is low-set with umbilical hernia, short edematous fingers without flexion creases, rocker-bottom feet, syndactyly of toes 2+3 bilaterally, and sacral meningocele. Internal examination (not illustrated) showed blood in the abdomen, subcapsular hemorrhage of the liver (measuring 40 × 23mm), partial malrotation of the gut, several accessory spleens, small adrenals, pleural and pericardial effusions, and an atrial septal defect.

Estimated developmental age: 21 weeks
Fertilization age: 23 weeks
Karyotype: 69,XXY

56

# CHAPTER 4

# Trisomy

Trisomy is the most common type of chromosome abnormality in spontaneous abortions. In our series of specimens examined pathologically, there were 622 specimens of nonmosaic autosomal trisomy, and eight cases with an additional sex chromosome, all XXY.

## Trisomy Types Among Abortions

Figure 4–1 illustrates the frequencies of trisomy for each chromosome in our total set of karyotyped spontaneous abortions (including those not evaluated pathologically). Trisomy was found for every chromosome except 1, 11, and 19. Trisomies 11 and 19 have been rarely found in other series, and by us once each in subsequent selected specimens. Trisomy 1 has never been found in a spontaneous abortion specimen but was found in a very early embryo after in vitro fertilization (Watt et al., 1987). Trisomy for chromosome 16 is by far the most common, making up 201/645 or 31% of all karyotyped autosomal trisomies in our series. This trisomy has never been reported in a full-term birth. In addition to the cases of nonmosaic trisomy, there were 60 cases of trisomy/normal mosaicism, 23 cases of double trisomy, and 12 cases of trisomy/double trisomy mosaicism. There were also 13 cases of hypertriploidy (70 chromosomes), 13 cases of hypertetraploidy (94 chromosomes), both of which probably result from a hyperhaploid gamete, and 11 cases in which trisomy was present along with another chromosomal anomaly such as monosomy X or a structural rearrangement. Thus a large proportion of what are usually grouped as "other" chromosome anomalies also include trisomy.

Because we examined 200 cases of trisomy 16, it can be meaningfully analyzed separately. The other trisomies can be usefully grouped into those that are often viable until birth (trisomies 13, 18, and 21), and the remainder, which are rarely or never seen at term (although the occasional mosaic case may survive). It should be remembered that even for those trisomies that we call "viable", the rate of loss during gestation is very high. From the frequencies of these trisomies in live-births and spontaneous abortions we can calculate that only about 30% of conceptions with trisomy 21 survive to birth. For conceptions with trisomy 18, this proportion decreases to about 5%, and it is even lower for trisomy 13.

Apparently no strong correlation exists between the frequency with which a particular trisomy is observed in spontaneous abortions and its ability to survive the gestational period. For instance, on the one hand the viable trisomies 21 and 13 are among the most common trisomies in spontaneous abortions (about 50 cases each in our series), but trisomies 15 and 22, which are nonviable, are just as common. On the other hand, trisomy 18, which is viable, occurred less often than such nonviable trisomies as 2 and 7.

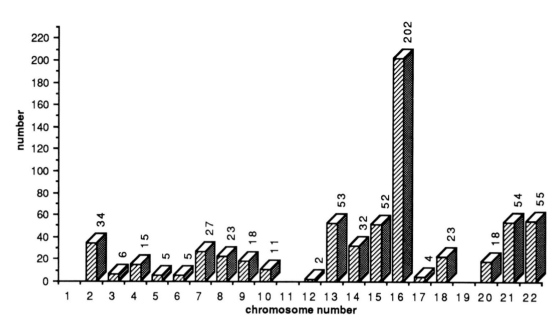

**Figure 4–1** Frequency of trisomy for each human chromosome among aborted specimens.

## Distribution of Specimen Classes

Table 4–1 shows the frequency of each morphological class by type of trisomy. Among conceptions with trisomy 16, 51% were received as placental fragments only. Among complete specimens almost half (47%) were intact empty sacs, and another 27% had minimal embryonic development, usually with a disorganized embryo almost directly attached to the amnion (Figs. 4–24 through 4–29). Only 26% of complete specimens had a well developed cord or embryo with cord (the largest of these was only 6 mm and macerated). All miscarriage series to date agree that only the most minimal embryonic development is associated with trisomy 16.

Among all other nonviable trisomic specimens, 42% were received as placental fragments only. Among complete specimens, 27% were intact empty sacs and 17% had minimal embryonic development, while 31% had a well developed cord, 23% an embryo, and 2% a fetus.

The four specimens which reached the fetal stage had trisomy 7, trisomy 15, trisomy 20, and trisomy 22. In the first three cases karyotypes were prepared from placental tissue because fetal tissue was too autolyzed for successful growth. The specimens with trisomy 20 (Fig. 4–41) and trisomy 15 were both apparently normal fetuses of 19-weeks developmental age. The possibility that the trisomy was confined to the placental tissues must be considered in these cases. The specimen with trisomy 7 was severely autolyzed, with a developmental age about 5 weeks behind gestational age and anomalies such as cleft palate, abnormal facies, and small kidneys and adrenals (Fig. 4–7). The fetus with trisomy 22 had both a fertilization and developmental age of 13 weeks, with a membranous ventricular septal defect, generalized edema, cystic hygromata, and abnormal facies (Fig. 4–56).

Among the nonviable trisomies there appeared to be some that have a greater potential for development:

**Table 4–1** Specimen Type Among Trisomies by Chromosome Number

| Chromosome number | Fragment | Intact empty sac | Disorganized embryo | Sac with cord | Embryo | Fetus | All specimens |
|---|---|---|---|---|---|---|---|
| 16 | 102 | 46 | 26 | 10 | 15 | 0 | 199 |
| % Of Complete Specimens | | 47.4 | 26.8 | 10.3 | 15.5 | 0 | (97) |
| **Nonviable** | | | | | | | |
| 1 | — | — | — | — | — | — | 0 |
| 2 | 16 | 14 | 0 | 2 | 2 | 0 | 34 |
| 3 | 3 | 2 | 1 | 0 | 0 | 0 | 6 |
| 4 | 4 | 0 | 6 | 3 | 1 | 0 | 14 |
| 5 | 3 | 1 | 0 | 0 | 1 | 0 | 5 |
| 6 | 1 | 4 | 0 | 0 | 0 | 0 | 5 |
| 7 | 12 | 6 | 2 | 3 | 2 | 1 | 26 |
| 8 | 14 | 5 | 1 | 1 | 1 | 0 | 22 |
| 9 | 11 | 1 | 2 | 3 | 1 | 0 | 22 |
| 10 | 4 | 2 | 3 | 2 | 0 | 0 | 11 |
| 11 | — | — | — | — | — | — | 0 |
| 12 | 1 | 1 | 0 | 0 | 0 | 0 | 2 |
| 14 | 15 | 0 | 2 | 5 | 7 | 0 | 29 |
| 15 | 11 | 3 | 3 | 26 | 6 | 1 | 50 |
| 17 | 0 | 1 | 2 | 1 | 0 | 0 | 4 |
| 19 | — | — | — | — | — | — | 0 |
| 20 | 10 | 3 | 1 | 0 | 3 | 1 | 18 |
| 22 | 20 | 3 | 7 | 7 | 16 | 1 | 54 |
| % Of Complete Specimens | | 26.6 | 17.3 | 30.6 | 23.1 | 2.3 | (173) |
| **Viable** | | | | | | | |
| 13 | 21 | 5 | 0 | 11 | 10 | 3 | 50 |
| 18 | 8 | 0 | 0 | 2 | 4 | 9 | 23 |
| 21 | 11 | 0 | 1 | 18 | 8 | 11 | 49 |
| % Of Complete Specimens | | 6.1 | 1.2 | 37.8 | 26.8 | 28.0 | (82) |

about half of complete specimens with trisomies 7, 8, 9, 14, 15, 20, and 22 had a well-developed cord and/or an embryo or fetus. Rare reports have been made of live-births with apparently nonmosaic trisomy for each of these chromosomes (Schinzel, 1984). The number of specimens of most of these trisomies is too few to make adequate comparisons with other series. Boué et al.

(1985) reported a greater capacity for development in certain trisomies such as 7–10 and 22. Creasy et al. (1976) reported a fetus with trisomy 22 in their series of banded karyotypes, and two fetuses with C-group trisomy in their unbanded series. Zerres et al. (1988) have also described the features of three embryos with trisomy 22.

To our knowledge only a few of the rudimentary embryos from nonviable trisomies have been studied histologically. Investigations by Kleinebrecht and Geisler (1975, 1984) and Geisler and Kleinebrecht (1978) of trisomy 2 and other chromosomally abnormal embryos, and by Ohama et al. (1977) of trisomy 17, confirmed the presence of rudimentary tissue organization in the growth-disorganized embryos which were studied. We also carried out histological examination of two specimens with trisomy 17 and found evidence of an apparent neural tube within the 2-mm embryonic remnant that was present.

Among viable trisomies 33% were received as placental fragments only (Table 4–1). In contrast to the nonviable trisomies, only 7% of complete specimens were intact empty sacs or small disorganized embryos: 38% had a well-developed cord with embryonic fragments, 27% were embryos, and 28% were fetuses over 30 mm. Fetuses were most common for trisomy 21, followed by trisomy 18, and then trisomy 13. Potential for viability during gestation follows the same order as does viability after birth. Figure 4–2 compares the morphological distributions for three classes of trisomy. The poor potential for development of trisomy 16 and other nonviable trisomies is clearly different than that for the viable trisomies.

Anomalies seen in spontaneously aborted embryos and fetuses with trisomy 13, 18, and 21 were consistent with the features found in full-term infants or electively terminated pregnancies where the fetus had these karyotypes (Moerman et al., 1988; Kinoshita et al., 1989).

Embryos or fetuses with trisomy 13 had midface hypoplasia with proboscis and cyclopia (Fig. 4–12), polydactyly, small adrenals, and cleft lip and palate. Boué et al. (1976) also reported an embryo with cyclocephaly, while the single case reported by Creasy et al. (1976) had only a cleft palate. Disruption of midface development leading to holoprosencephaly, synophthalmia,

Figure 4–2 Distribution of types of trisomy among each morphological class of specimens.

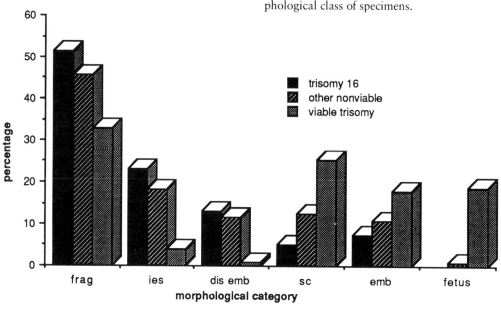

dysgenesis of teeth, cleft lip, cardiovascular malformations, and other anomalies are common (Sperber et al., 1989).

Embryos and fetuses with trisomy 18 had omphalocele, (Figs. 4–35 and 4–39), nuchal hygromata (Fig. 4–35), cleft lip and palate (Fig. 4–36), heart defects, polydactyly (Figs. 4–34 and 4–39), and kidney anomalies and prune belly (Figs. 4–38 and 4–39). Two embryos with trisomy 18 reported by Lauritsen (1976) were stated to have anencephaly, while Creasy et al. (1976) described one apparently normal fetus and one with only talipes. Prune belly arising from prostatic hypoplasia has been reported in fetuses with trisomy 18 (Hoagland et al., 1988). Cystic hygromata have been reported in fetuses with trisomies 18 and 21 (Chervenak et al., 1983).

Specimens with trisomy 21 usually appeared quite normal, but shortening of the upper arms and legs was noted in larger fetuses (Figs. 4–47 through 4–50). The presence of shortened femurs has now been documented in Down syndrome fetuses in utero by ultrasound by Benacerraf et al. (1987) and Lockwood et al. (1987a), although its use as a diagnostic tool is doubtful (Peters, 1989). One embryo, with trisomy 21 resulting from a translocation, was severely malformed with an encephalocele and cleft lip (Fig. 4–43). In general we did not find more severe anomalies in the spontaneously aborted specimens with trisomy 21 than were found by those who have examined specimens of induced abortions after prenatal diagnosis (Gullotta et al. 1981).

## Gestational Age at Abortion

The mean gestations for abortions with trisomy 16, other nonviable trisomies, and viable trisomies were 11.7 weeks, 12.1 weeks, and 13.1 weeks, respectively. The distributions of gestational age are not very different for the viable and nonviable trisomies, with the modal time of expulsion being between 77 and 84 days in each case. However, 21/120 or 18% of viable trisomies were retained beyond 16 weeks of gestation, while only 35/491 or 7% of nonviable trisomies (including trisomy 16) were retained this long. Of the 21 viable trisomies, 16 were trisomy 21, four were trisomy 18, and only one was trisomy 13. The correlation between viability and gestation at abortion is not nearly so clear as that for degree of development achieved, reflecting the fact that many pregnancies are retained long after development has stopped. Among trisomy 16 pregnancies, while gestation according to LMP ranged up to 24 weeks, development never exceeded a rudimentary embryo. The trisomy 16 case with the longest gestational age was an intact empty sac with no visible embryo when expelled.

## Maternal Age

Maternal age for trisomies was elevated when compared with that of livebirths of the same time period, or with chromosomally normal spontaneous abortions. In general the mean maternal age increases with decreasing size of the chromosome which is trisomic (Table 4–2). Mean age for pregnancies with trisomy 16 was 29.4, while for pregnancies with trisomy 14–22 it was 33.

Table 4–2 Maternal Age of Trisomic Spontaneous Abortions

| Trisomy | Number of Cases | Mean Maternal Age |
|---|---|---|
| 2–6 | 65 | 26.8 ± 0.9 |
| 6–12 | 81 | 30.3 ± 0.8 |
| 13 | 53 | 30.8 ± 0.8 |
| 14–15 | 85 | 32.6 ± 1.2 |
| 16 | 200 | 29.4 ± 0.4 |
| 18 | 23 | 33.6 ± 1.5 |
| 17, 20 | 22 | 33.9 ± 2.1 |
| 21 | 53 | 33.2 ± 1.0 |
| 22 | 55 | 33.5 ± 0.8 |
| Livebirths | | 26.5 ± 0.5 |

Pregnancies with trisomies 2–6 had a mean maternal age of 26.8, which is not elevated above that for livebirths.

### Chorionic Villi

In the cases of trisomy 16 where villi were classified morphologically, 53% had villi described as normal or clubbed, 30% were described as cystic, and 16% were described as hypoplastic. One specimen was classified as a hydatidiform mole. Among other trisomies, 60% had normal or clubbed villi, 16% were cystic, 24% hypo-plastic, and there was one specimen described as a mole. There was a significant trend for the specimens with hypoplastic villi to have longer gestations than those with other villi types, and, as a result, specimens with viable trisomies had a much higher proportion of hypoplastic villi (40%) than those with nonviable trisomies (18%). It should be noted that this association with increasing gestation in the pregnancies with hypoplastic villi was *not* observed in the cases with monosomy X where this villus type was so frequent. Philippe, Boué (1969), and Honoré et al. (1976) have also commented on the hypoplasia in trisomic placentas.

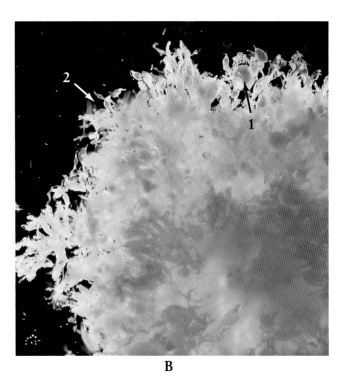

B

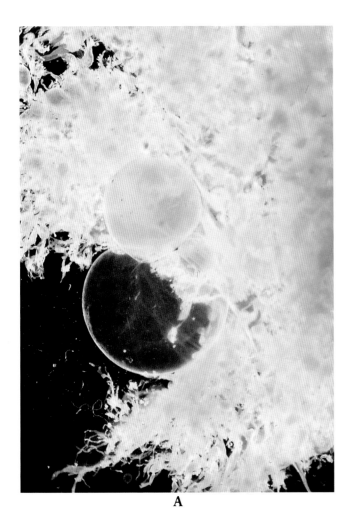

A

**Figure 4–3** (4596) (**A**) The only evidence of embryonic development is apparent twin chorionic sacs. (**B**) Abundant villous development, showing mixed pattern of cystic (1) and clubbed (2) villi.

Fertilization age: 9 weeks
 Karyotype: 47,XX,+2

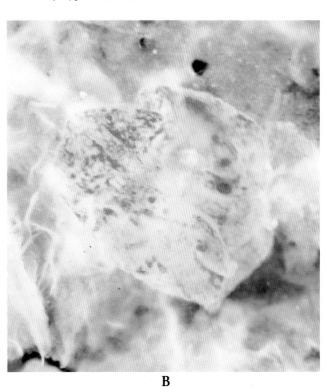

B

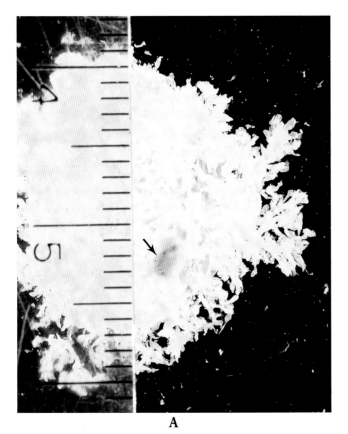

A

**Figure 4–4** (4650) (**A**) Intact empty chorionic sac, 20 mm in diameter, covered with villi. Note the yolk sac (arrow). (**B**) Close-up of yolk sac showing fetal blood islands. No fetal blood vessels can be seen within the villi.

Fertilization age: 42 days
 Karyotype: 47,XX,+3

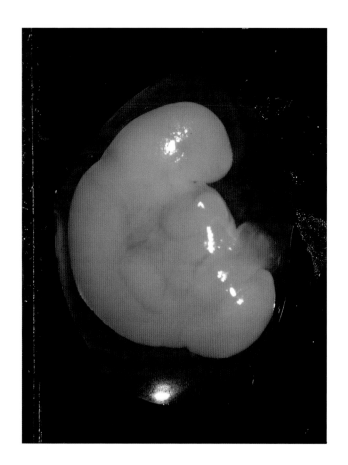

**Figure 4–5** (2868) Autolyzed embryo attached to amnion (8-mm CRL). Heart prominence visible, no eyes seen.

Estimated developmental age: 35 days
Fertilization age: 49 days
Karyotype: 47,XX,+4.

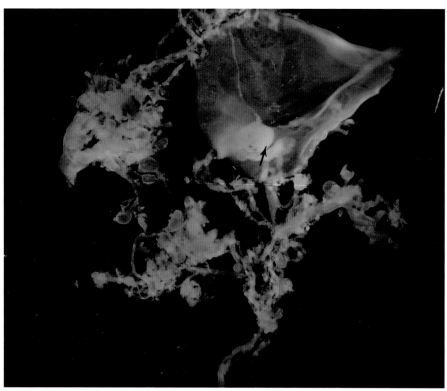

**Figure 4–6** (3535) Embryo attached directly to amnion, two pigmented eyespots visible (arrow). Mixed pattern of cystic and hypoplastic villi.

Fertilization age: unknown
Karyotype: 47,XY,+7

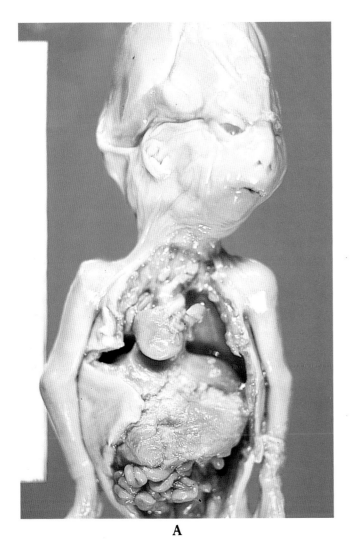

A

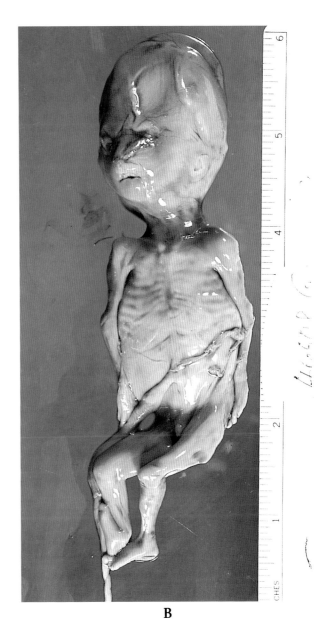

B

**Figure 4–7** (1536) (**A** and **B**) A 100-mm CRL, 43 g, severely autolysed male fetus with abnormal facies, small chin, cleft palate, micropenis, single umbilical artery, small kidneys and adrenals, right descending aorta and malrotation. (Byrne et al., 1985; Byrne, 1983; Byrne and Blanc, 1985.)

Estimated developmental age: 13 weeks
Fertilization age: 18 weeks
Karyotype: 47,XY,+7

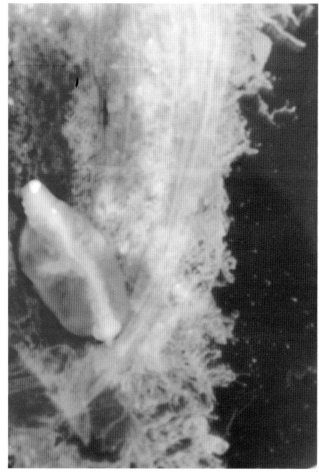

A

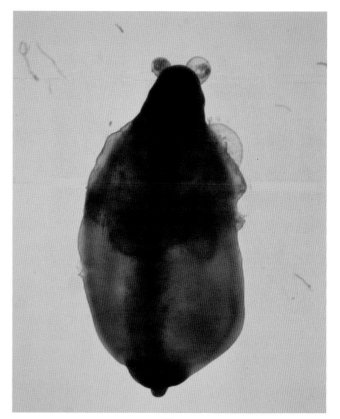

B

**Figure 4–8** (4493) (**A**) Embryo in original position attached to sac. (**B**) Close-up of embryo, 11-mm CRL, showing numerous dilatations at head end and dilated flank region.

Fertilization age: 71 days
    Karyotype: 47,XX,+8

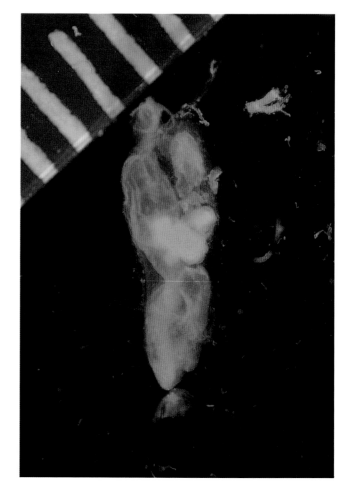

**Figure 4–9** (3405) Uterine cast contained intact sac (30 × 20 mm) with this 3-mm disorganized embryo in a ruptured 5-mm diameter amniotic sac.

Fertilization age: unknown
    Karyotype: 47,XY,+9

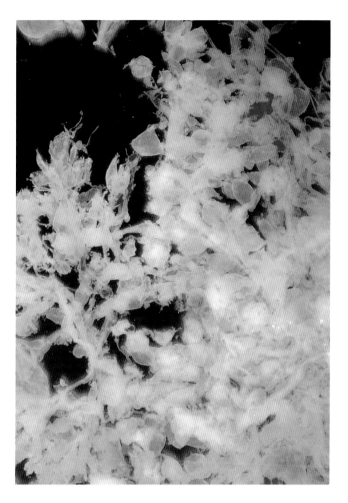

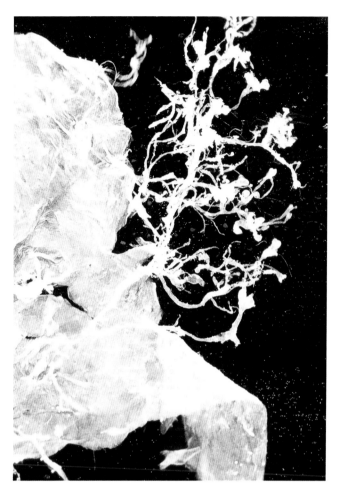

**Figure 4–10** (4431) Abundant villous development with some cysts visible. Original specimen was an intact empty sac with no evidence of embryonic development. The fragments of bloody tissue are probably maternal decidua.

Fertilization age: 81 days
    Karyotype: 47,XY,+10

**Figure 4–11** (4602) Hypoplastic villi branching from maternal surface of chorionic sac. Some evidence of terminal swelling—"clubbing".

Fertilization age: 102 days
    Karyotype: 47,XY,+10

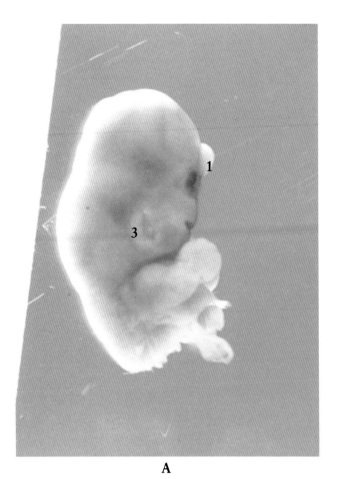

**A**

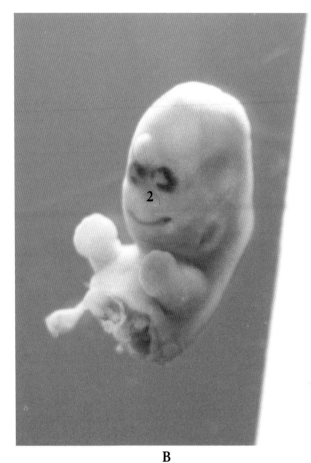

**B**

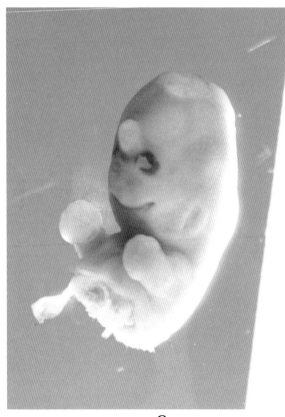

**C**

**Figure 4–12** (1634) (**A** and **B**) A 13-mm fragment of upper part of autolyzed embryo showing proboscis (1), extreme hypotelorism with bilateral colobomata (2), and auricular hillocks (3). (**C**) Digital rays and patches visible on hands. Limb development appears retarded for the size of the embryo. (Byrne et al., 1985)

Estimated developmental age: 49–51 days
Fertilization age: 64 days
Karyotype: 47,XX,+13

68

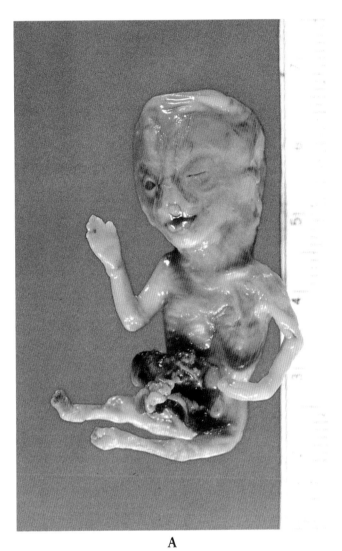

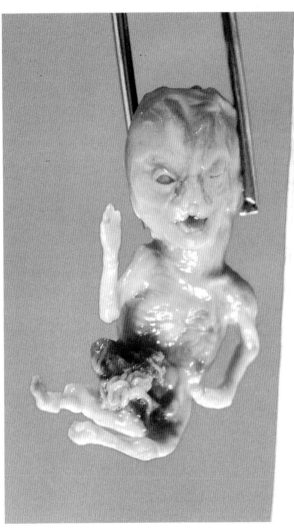

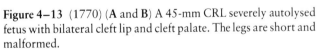

A                                                        B

**Figure 4–13** (1770) (**A** and **B**) A 45-mm CRL severely autolysed fetus with bilateral cleft lip and cleft palate. The legs are short and malformed.

Estimated developmental age: 10 weeks
Fertilization age: 13 weeks
Karyotype: 47,XY,+13

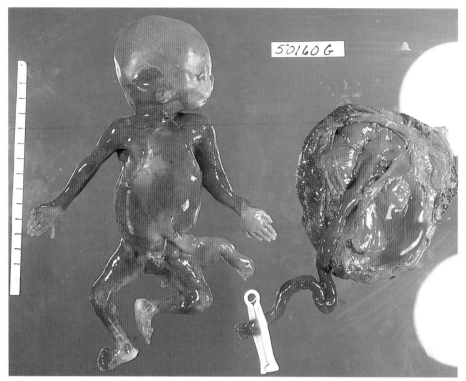

**A**

**Figure 4–14** (50160) Induced abortion following saline instillation. (**A**) A 163-mm CRL male fetus with abnormally shaped skull, low-set ears, micrognathia, and polydactyly. (**B**) Symmetrical postaxial polydactyly of both hands and feet. (**C**) Thoracic dissection showing blunted apex of heart due to abnormal blood flow because of atrial septal defect. Ductus arteriosus enters aortic arch directly opposite exit of left carotid artery (arrow). (**D**) Adrenal, small relative to kidney (arrows).

Estimated developmental age: 18 weeks
Fertilization age: 18 weeks
Karyotype: 47,XY,+13

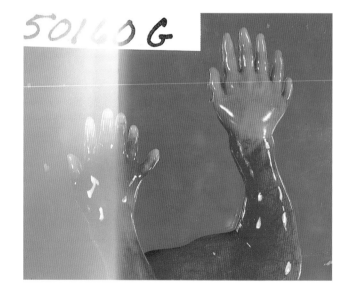

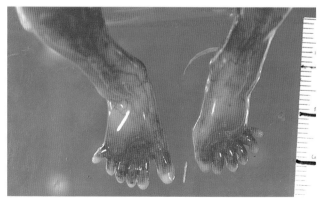

**B**

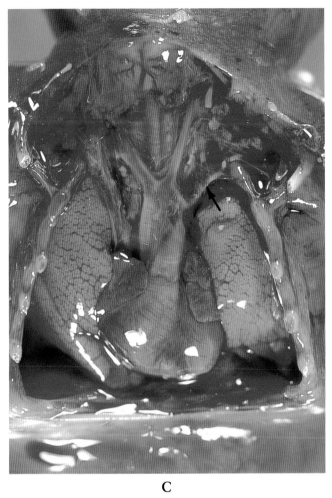

C

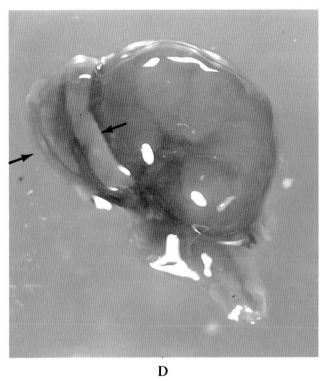

D

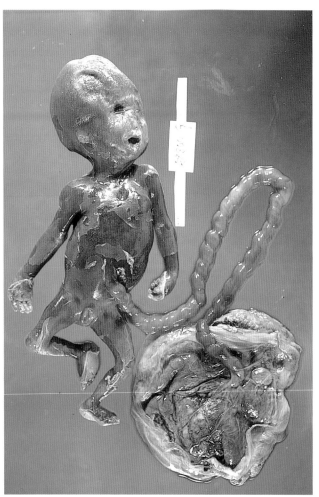

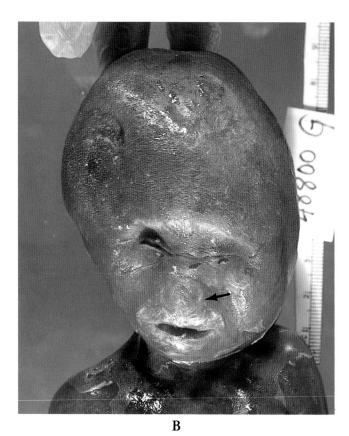

B

A

**Figure 4–15** (48800) Induced saline abortion. A 192-mm CRL, 372 g male fetus. (**A** and **B**) Note midline hypoplasia with confluent eyebrows, microphthalmia, and hypotelorism. The nose is very flattened with one nonpatent naris (arrow). The mouth is small and the jaw is narrow. The penis and the feet are both small, the right foot is clubbed. Dissection revealed normal lungs, liver, adrenals, and kidneys. The heart has a dysplastic aortic valve, and an atrial septal defect (septum secundum type?).

Estimated developmental age: 19 weeks
                Fertilization age: 19 weeks
                         Karyotype: 47,XY,+13

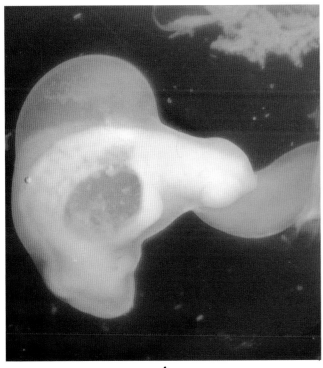

A

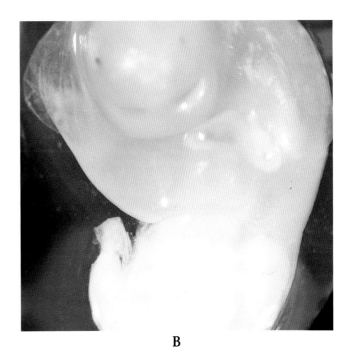

B

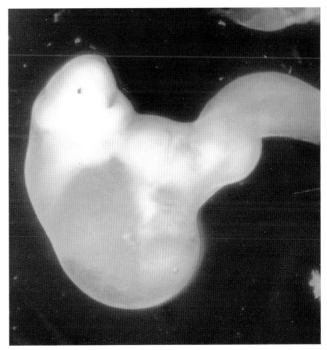

C

**Figure 4–16** (864769) (**A** and **B**) Embryo (unknown CRL) in amnion. (**C**) Note eyes, mouth, and heart prominence.

Estimated developmental age: 26 days
Fertilization age: unknown
Karyotype: 47,XX,+14

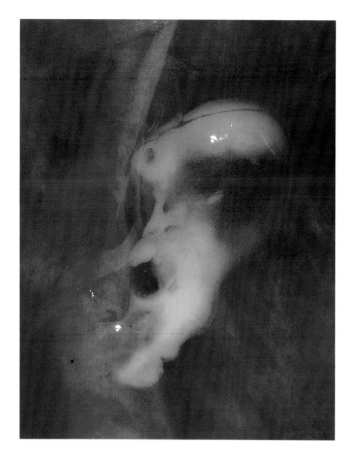

Figure 4–17 (2871) A 5-mm embryo received in an intact sac, connected by a short 1-mm body stalk. Note the brain. An eye, upper limb bud, and somites are visible.

Estimated developmental age: cannot be estimated
Fertilization age: 57 days
Karyotype: 47,XY,+14

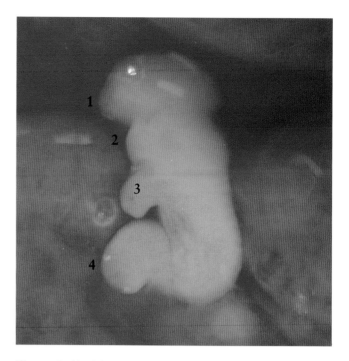

Figure 4–18 (2853) A 5-mm CRL embryo. Note forebrain prominence (1), mandibular arch (2), heart prominence (3), and body stalk (4). (Byrne, 1983.)

Estimated developmental age: 28 days
Fertilization age: 68 days
Karyotype: 47,XY,+14

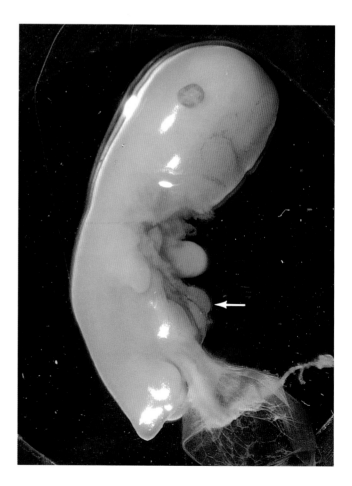

Figure 4–19 (2940) A 19-mm CRL embryo received in intact sac, attached by short 1-mm cord. Autolysis probably accounts for loss of cervical flexure and rupture at heart prominence (arrow). Paddle-shaped upper limb, pigmented eye spot. An encephalocele present in the occipital region cannot be seen in this photograph. (Byrne and Warburton, 1986; Byrne et al., 1985.)

Estimated developmental age: 37–43 days
Fertilization age: 42 days
Karyotype: 46,XY,−13,+t(13q14q)

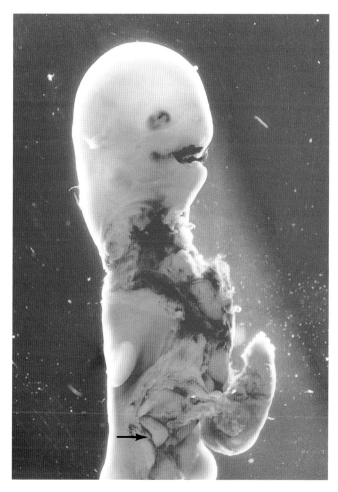

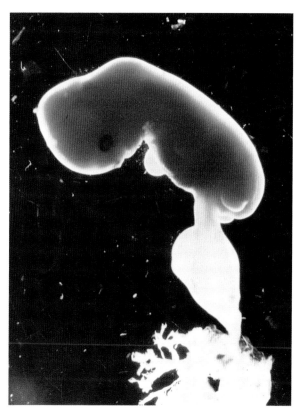

**Figure 4–20** (4631) A 17-mm CRL autolysed and partially dissected embryo. Note pigmented eye with physiological (?) coloboma, paddle-shaped upper and lower limbs without digital rays, gonad in right pelvis (arrow).

Estimated developmental age: 37–43 days
Fertilization age: 85 days
Karyotype: 47,XX,+14

**Figure 4–21** (4548) A 15-mm CRL embryo, attached to sac by 10-mm cord with lateral dilatation. The embryo appears normally developed, with eyes, mouth, and upper and lower limbs.

Estimated developmental age: 44–46 days
Fertilization age: 65 days
Karyotype: 47,XY,+14

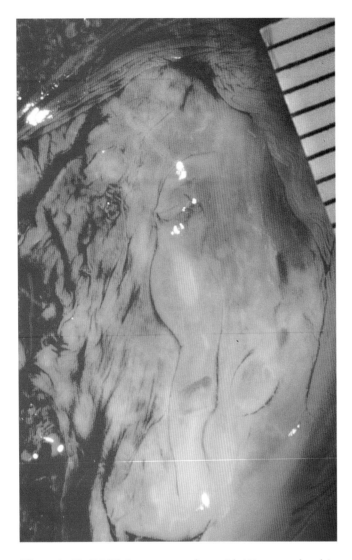

**Figure 4–22** (2282) Large ruptured sac with 15-mm cord and 4-mm brown mass of autolysed fetal tissue at the free end.

Fertilization age: 104 days
    Karyotype: 47,XY,+15

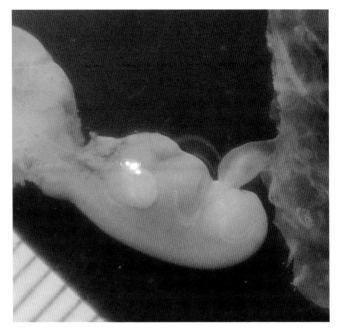

**Figure 4–23** (2254) A 17-mm CRL embryo, apparently normal, received in an intact sac. Pigmented eye spots are not visible in this photograph. Note paddle-shaped upper limb while lower extremities are still at the limb bud stage; 4-mm cord with dilatation.

Estimated developmental age: 37–43 days
    Fertilization age: 62 days
        Karyotype: 47,XY,+15

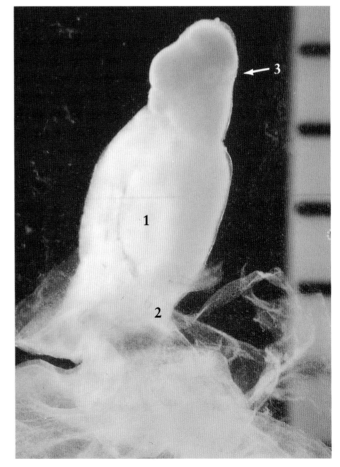

**Figure 4–24** (1839) A 4-mm CRL disorganized embryo (1) attached directly to amnion (2), no cord visible. No limb buds seen. Note cephalic end with unpigmented eye spot (3).

Fertilization age: 60 days
    Karyotype: 47,XY,+16

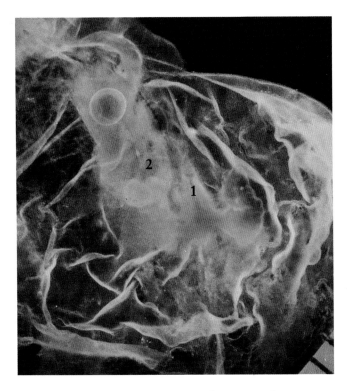

**Figure 4–25** (2286) Amnion, 20-mm diameter, with structures, probably representing aberrant yolk sac (1) and embryo (2).

Fertilization age: unknown
    Karyotype: 47,XX,+16

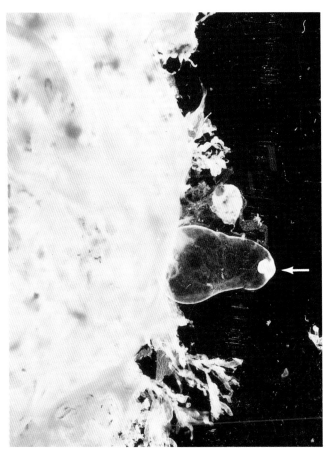

**Figure 4–27** (4622) Amniotic sac projecting out from chorion with disorganized embryo attached directly to amnion on extreme right (arrow).

Fertilization age: 49 days
    Karyotype: 47,XY,+16

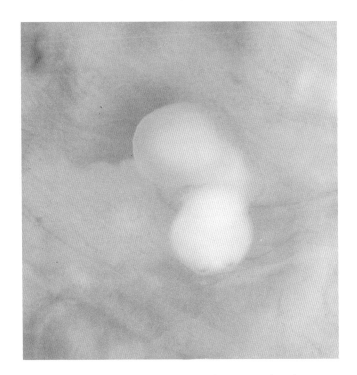

**Figure 4–26** (2029) A 1-mm CRL disorganized embryo, attached directly to amnion. No cord is visible. No embryonic structures can be identified.

Fertilization age: 12 weeks
    Karyotype: 47,XX,+16

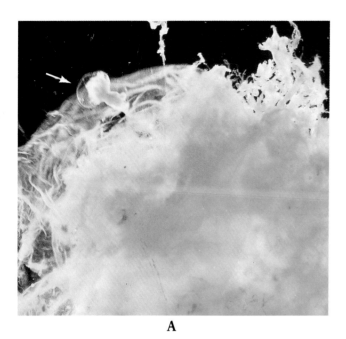

A

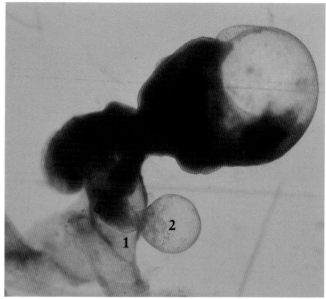

B

**Figure 4–28** (4594) (**A**) A 3-mm severely disorganized embryo (arrow) attached to surface of amnion. (**B**) Close-up of embryo showing edematous head, umbilical cord stump (1) and yolk sac (?) (2).

Fertilization age: 46 days
  Karyotype: 47,XX,+16

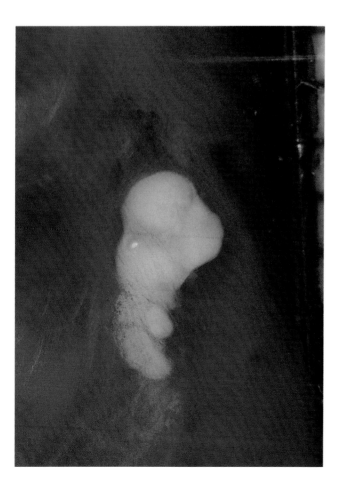

**Figure 4–29** (2933) A 3-mm CRL disorganized embryo, head end and upper limb bud visible. Received in intact amnion (8-mm diameter) within a large chorion without villi on its maternal surface.

Fertilization age: 9 weeks
  Karyotype: 47,XX,+16

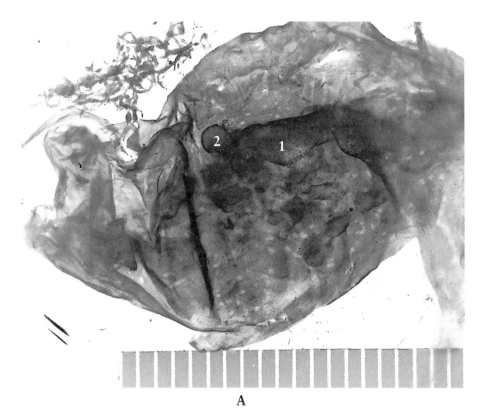

**A**

**Figure 4–30** (1737) (A) Free amniotic sac 20 mm in diameter containing 13 × 2-mm cord (1) with a 2-mm nubbin of embryo (2) at one end. (B) Disorganized embryo. Two eye spots may be present.

Fertilization age: 10 weeks
　　Karyotype: 47,XX,+17

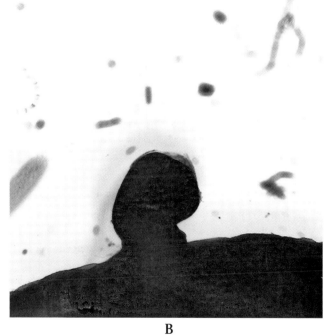

**B**

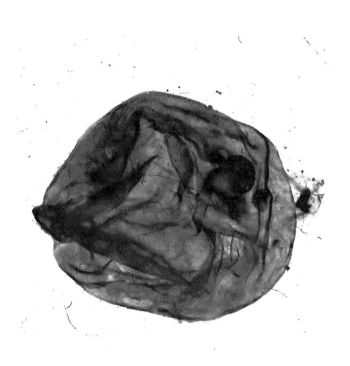

**Figure 4–31** (1809) A 2-mm disorganized embryo connected directly to the surface of a 9-mm diameter intact amnion.

Fertilization age: 58 days
　　Karyotype: 47,XY,+17

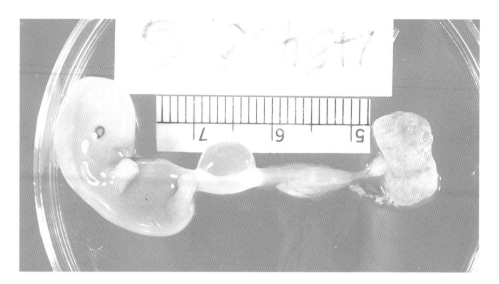

**Figure 4–32** (1252) A 23-mm CRL slightly autolysed embryo received in an intact sac. Digital rays formed anteriorly; only digital notches are present on posterior limb buds. Note dilatations on cord; villi cystic (up to 1 mm).

Estimated developmental age: 50–51 days
Fertilization age: 79 days
Karyotype: 47,XY,+18

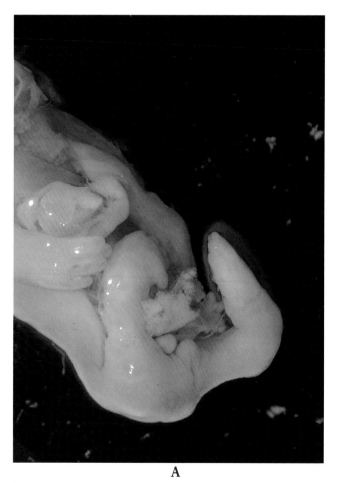

**A**

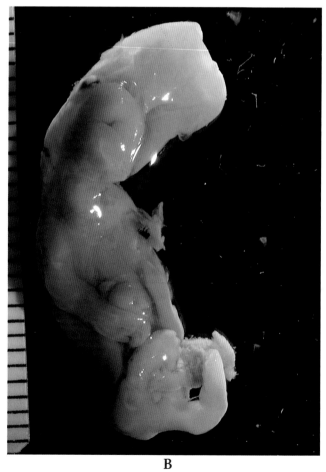

**B**

**Figure 4–33** (2844) A 31-mm CRL severely autolysed fetus, with skull collapsed. (**A**) Note indeterminate external genitalia, and abnormal position of legs. (**B**) Oral cleft is visible.

Estimated developmental age: 8 weeks
Fertilization age: 13 weeks
Karyotype: 47,XY,+18

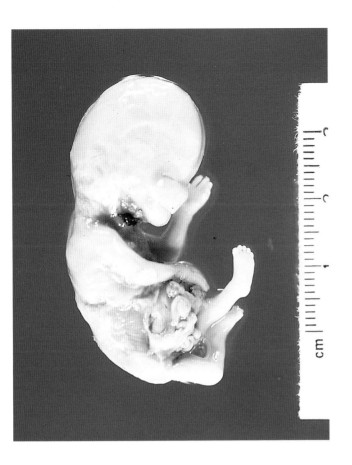

**Figure 4–34** (3131) A 38-mm CRL fetus, severely autolysed. Abdominal wall disintegrating and viscera protruding. Polydactyly of both hands.

Estimated developmental age: 8–9 weeks
Fertilization age: 13 weeks
Karyotype: 47,XY,+18/48,XY,+2,+18

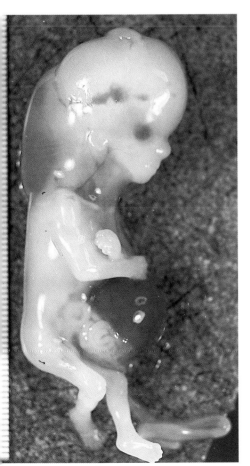

A

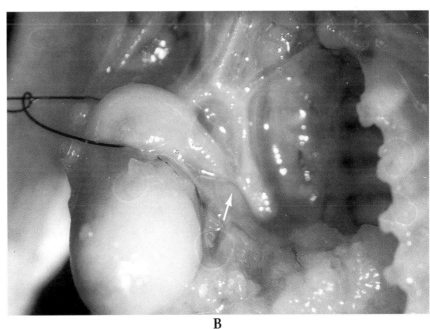

B

**Figure 4–35** (1215) (**A**) A 55-mm CRL well-preserved fetus with omphalocele, and nuchal hygroma; normal male genitalia externally and internally. (**B**) Heart deflected to the right, to show the very narrow opening of the ductus arteriosus into the descending aorta (arrow). (Byrne and Warburton, 1979; Byrne, 1985.)

Estimated developmental age: 9 weeks
Fertilization age: 11 weeks
Karyotype: 47,XY,+18

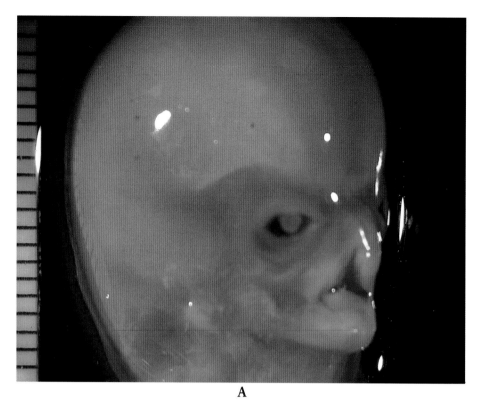

A

**Figure 4–36** (2418) (**A**) A 55-mm somewhat autolysed fetus with cleft lip and palate. (**B**) Normal female genitalia: ovary (1), uterus (2), single umbilical artery, right only (3). (Byrne, 1983; Byrne and Blanc, 1985; Byrne et al., 1985.)

Estimated developmental age: 9–10 weeks
Fertilization age: unknown
Karyotype: 47,XX,+18

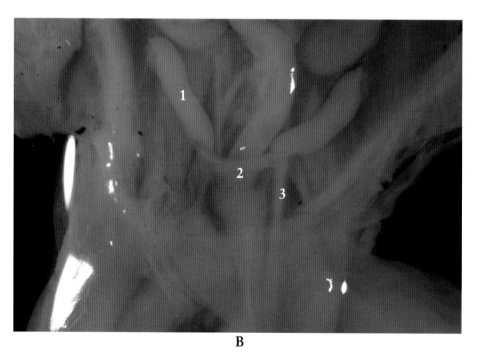

B

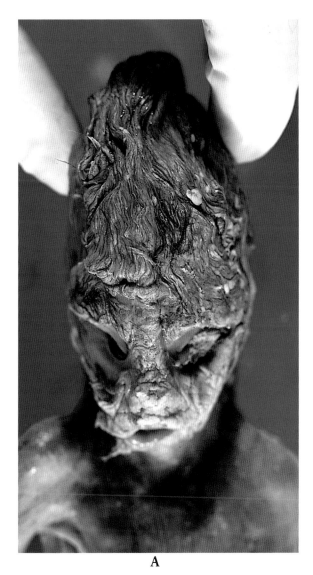

A

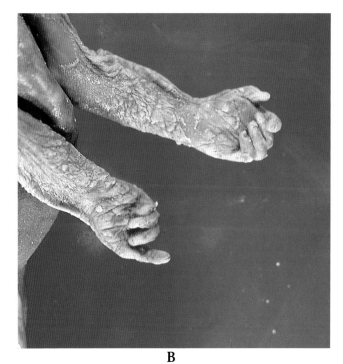

B

C

Figure 4–37 (50239) One of twins, delivered at 34 weeks: normal twin born alive, the other shown here died in utero at approximately 21 weeks. (A) A 186-mm CRL female fetus, severely autolysed, skull collapsed. (B) Abnormally positioned fingers, typical of trisomy 18 with lowset short thumbs. Note extensive deposition of white vernix on skin. (C) Membranous ventricular septal defect. The lungs were hypoplastic.

Estimated developmental age: 21 weeks
Fertilization age: 34 weeks
Karyotype: 47,XX,+18

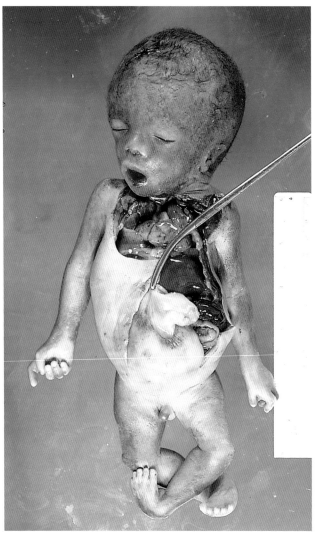

A

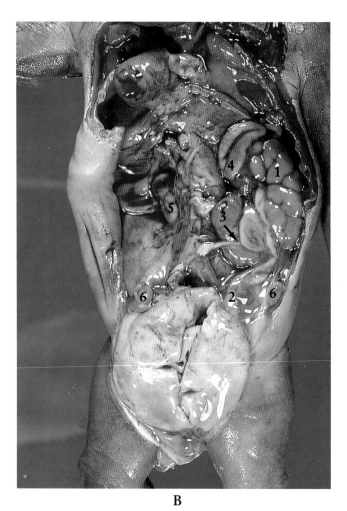

B

**Figure 4–38** (1541) A 210-mm CRL well-preserved male fetus. (**A**) Note small abnormal face, clenched fists, slack skin in abdomen (prune belly), small scrotum and penis. There are no flexion creases on the terminal phalanges of any fingers. The femur is short, and the hips do not flex. There is severe clubbed foot, with syndactyly between toes 3 and 4 on both feet. (**B**) Thoracic and abdominal dissection revealed enormously enlarged and fibrosed urinary bladder as the probable cause of the prune belly. No distal obstruction could be found. The kidneys (1) were fused, with pronounced fetal folds. The left ureter is enlarged (2), and the right is atrophic (3). The left adrenal (4) is normal; the right (5) is also normally positioned and shaped. The testes are normal (6). (Byrne and Blanc, 1985; Byrne et al., 1985.)

Estimated developmental age: 23 weeks
Fertilization age: 25 weeks
Karyotype: 47,XY,+18

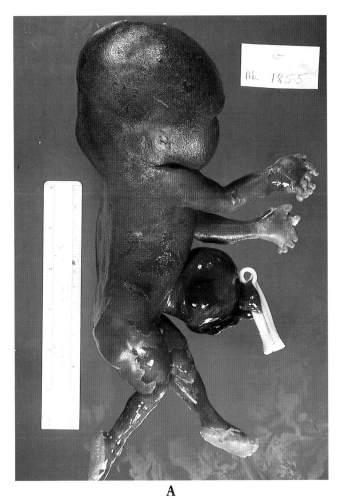

A

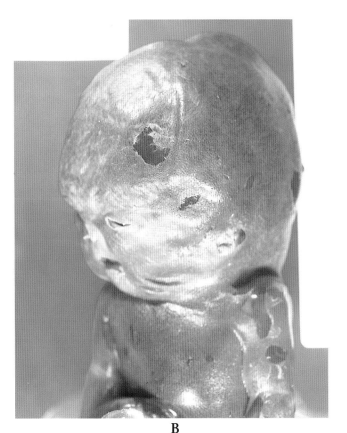

B

**Figure 4–39** (1855) (**A** and **B**) A 192-mm slightly autolysed male fetus, weight 585 g. External malformations noted are macrocephaly, (hydrocephalus ?), microphthalmia, hypertelorism, low-set hypoplastic ears with abnormal helix, micrognathia, high-arched palate, small mouth, small and flattened nose, omphalocele, bilateral syndactyly of hands and feet, polydactyly of the hands, and clubfeet. Internally the lungs were hypoplastic, and there were bilateral pleural effusions; the heart was enlarged with a ventricular septal defect. Also noted were accessory pancreas and spleen, left renal agenesis, hypoplasia of the diaphragm, malrotation of the gut, and single umbilical artery. (Byrne et al., 1985; Byrne and Blanc, 1985.)

Estimated developmental age: 26 weeks
Fertilization age: 26 weeks
Karyotype: 47,XY,+18

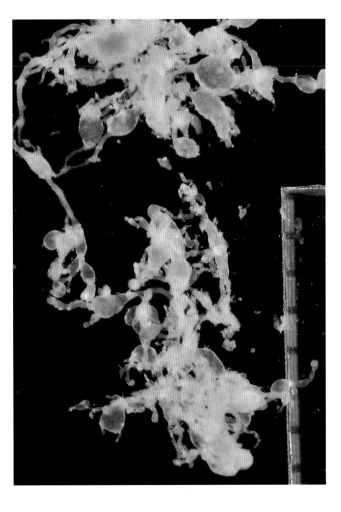

**Figure 4–40** (1970) Clubbed and cystic villi. Specimen was a ruptured sac without cord attachment site. No embryo was present.

Fertilization age: 11 weeks
Karyotype: 47,XX,+20

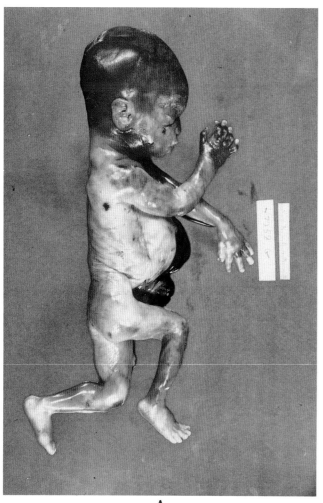

A

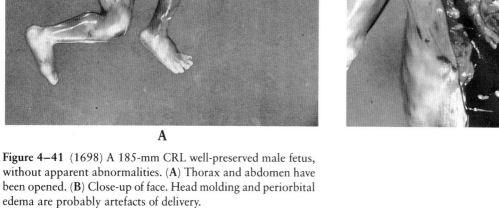

B

**Figure 4–41** (1698) A 185-mm CRL well-preserved male fetus, without apparent abnormalities. (**A**) Thorax and abdomen have been opened. (**B**) Close-up of face. Head molding and periorbital edema are probably artefacts of delivery.

Estimated developmental age: 19 weeks
Fertilization age: unknown
Karyotype: 47,XY,+20

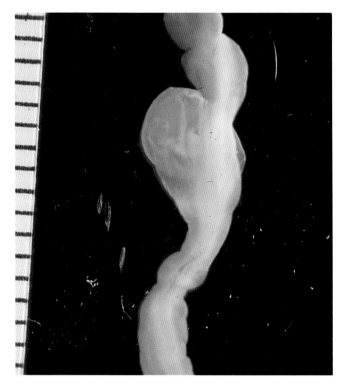

**Figure 4–42** (2065) Fragment of cord with 2-mm piece of embryonic tissue, received in a ruptured sac. Note cystic dilatations on cord. Villi were hypoplastic.

Fertilization age: 81 days
    Karyotype: 47,XY,+21

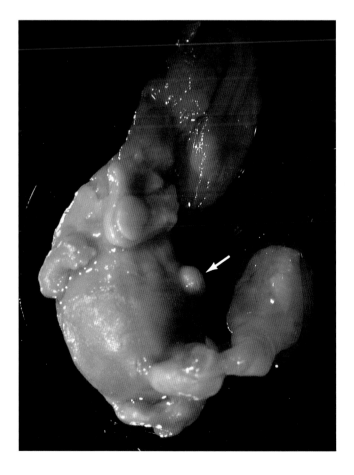

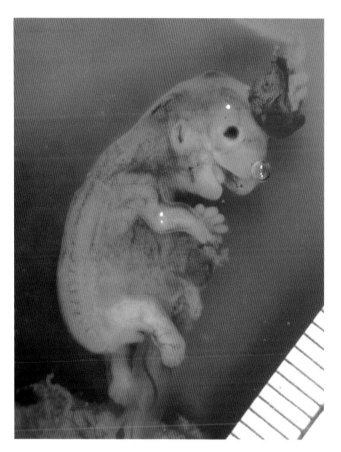

**Figure 4–43** (2617) A 24-mm well-preserved embryo with cleft lip and coronal exencephalus with herniated meninges and brain tissue; note abnormal profile and large abdomen. (Byrne, 1983; Byrne & Warburton, 1986; Byrne et al., 1985.)

Estimated developmental age: 53–54 days
    Fertilization age: 49 days
        Karyotype: 46,XY,−21,+t(21q21q)

**Figure 4–44** (2822) A 24-mm CRL severely autolysed fixed embryo; head collapsed. Left upper limb reduced to a rounded stump (arrow), right hand seems normal with digital rays. Lower limbs are rudimentary and fused together (sirenomelia). Cord with cystic dilatations. (Byrne et al., 1985.)

Estimated developmental age: 53–54 days
    Fertilization age: 17 weeks
        Karyotype: 47,XY,+21

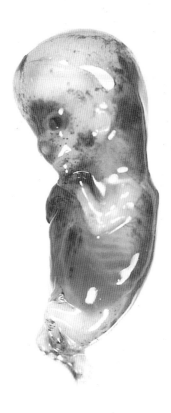

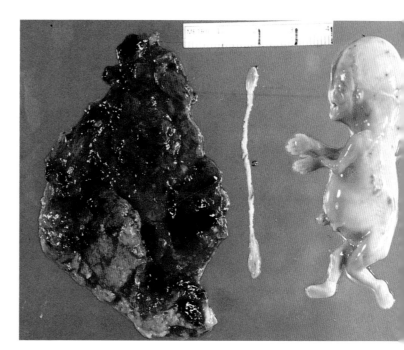

**Figure 4–46** (2581) A 58-mm CRL severely autolysed female fetus with dysmorphic facies, short nose, pointed chin, and intestines protruding through ruptured abdominal wall. Short cord, very thin and twisted. No internal anomalies. Short arms and legs, particularly humerus and femur. Suggestion of nuchal hygroma. (Byrne et al., 1985.)

Estimated developmental age: 9–10 weeks
Fertilization age: 14 weeks
Karyotype:47,XX,+21

**Figure 4–45** (3051) A 33-mm CRL well-preserved fetus with short arms and legs. No other apparent abnormalities.

Estimated developmental age: 8 weeks
Fertilization age: 53 days
Karyotype: 47,XY,+21

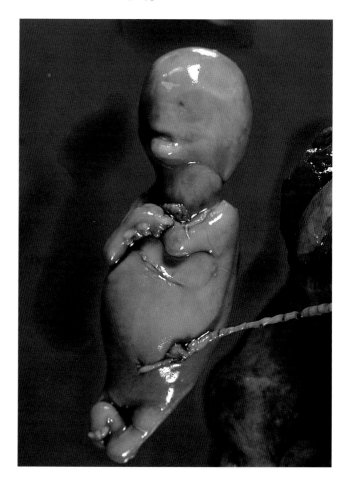

**Figure 4–47** (2607) A 55-mm CRL female, severely autolysed with dysmorphic facies and pointed chin. Protruding abdomen. Arms and legs abnormally positioned, and severely contracted, with webbing (pterygium) at axillae of arms. Arms and legs short. No internal anomalies. Cord short and twisted.

Estimated developmental age: 9–10 weeks
Fertilization age: 19 weeks
Karyotype: 47,XX,+21

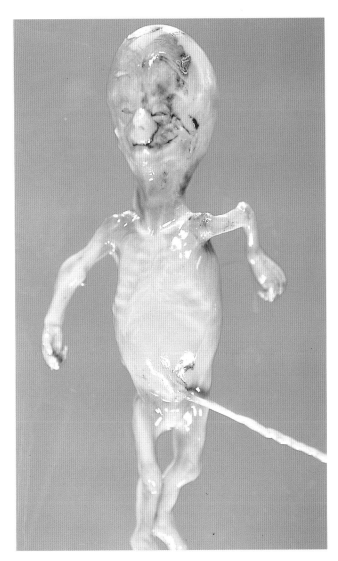

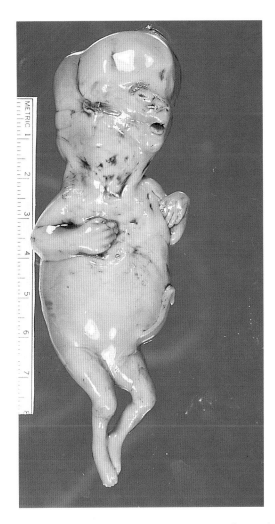

**Figure 4–49** (1145) A 75-mm CRL severely autolysed female fetus, quite edematous; abdomen distended, short arms and legs. Malrotation of the gut was present.

Estimated development age: 11 weeks
Fertilization age: 18 weeks
Karyotype: 47,XX,+21

**Figure 4–48** (2904) A 65-mm CRL severely autolysed female fetus with dysmorphic face and pointed chin. Short humerus and femur. No internal anomalies.

Estimated development age: 10 weeks
Fertilization age: unknown
Karyotype: 46,XX,−21,+t(21q21q)

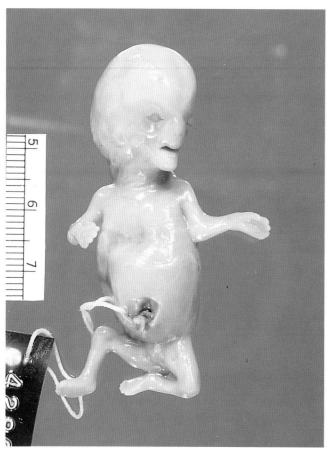

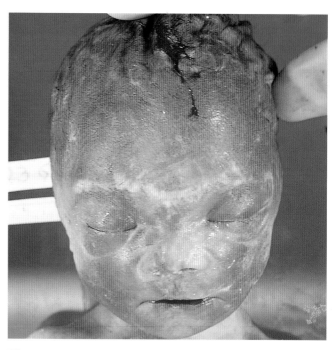

**Figure 4–51** (951) A 242-mm well-preserved female fetus with probable hypertelorism. There was a simian crease on the left hand, and a membranous ventricular septal defect. (Byrne and Warburton, 1979; Byrne et al., 1985.)

Estimated developmental age: 25 weeks
Fertilization age: 18 weeks (sic)
Karyotype: 47,XX,+21

**Figure 4–50** (784) A 75-mm CRL severely autolysed female fetus with dysmorphic facies and pointed chin; protruding abdomen, short arms and legs. Photographed after fixation.

Estimated developmental age: 11 weeks
Fertilization age: 12 weeks
Karyotype: 47,XY,+21

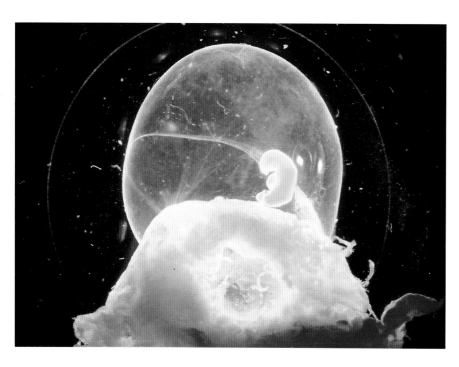

**Figure 4–52** (1336) A 3-mm embryo attached directly to sac 13 mm in diameter. Limb buds and tail are present.

Estimated developmental age: 28 days
Fertilization age: 55 days
Karyotype: 47,XX,+22

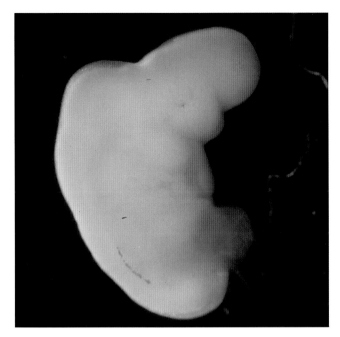

**Figure 4–53** (2996) A 5-mm CRL embryo with umbilical stump visible but no eyes or limb buds visible.

Estimated developmental age: 26 days
Fertilization age: 68 days
Karyotype: 47,XY,+22

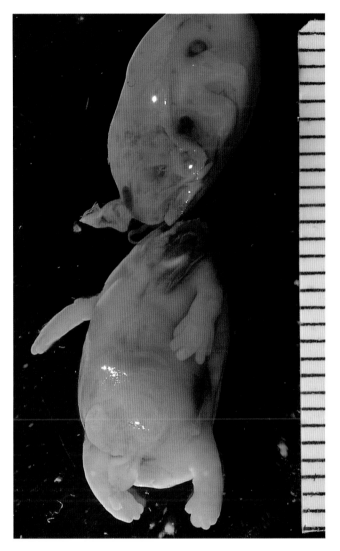

**Figure 4–55** (2851) A 22-mm total CRL severely autolysed embryo received in two fragments. Some area of old hemorrhage around the site of rupture. Palate not yet fused. Sex indeterminate. Digits on upper limbs well formed. Suggestion of syndactyly between digits 2 and 3.

Estimated developmental age: 49–51 days
Fertilization age: 11 weeks
Karyotype: 47,XY,+22

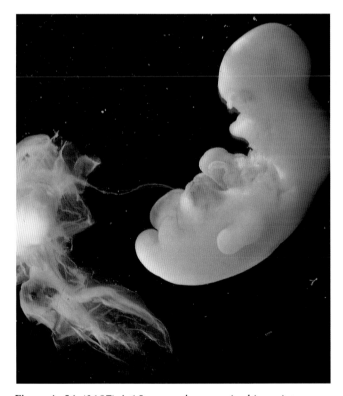

**Figure 4–54** (3197) A 15-mm embryo received in an intact amniotic sac. Embryo is quite autolysed with rupture at neck region. Head abnormally shaped. Eyespot is barely visible, and limbs are paddle shaped indicating retarded development relative to CRL.

Estimated developmental age: 44–46 days
Fertilization age: 63 days
Karyotype: 47,XY,+22

91

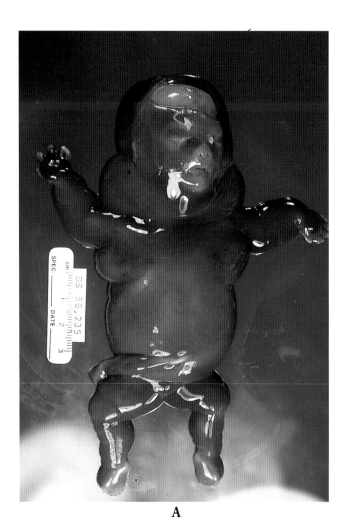

**A**

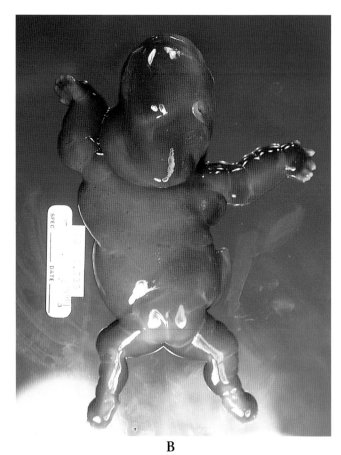

**B**

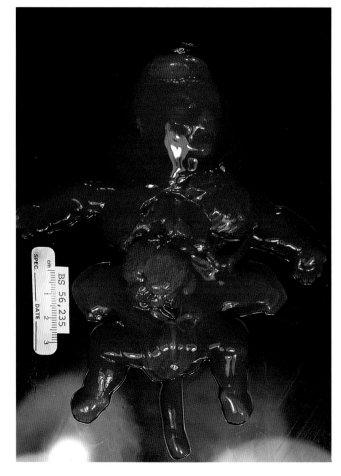

**Figure 4–56** (3758) (**A** and **B**) A 110-mm CRL female fetus with generalized edema, cystic hygroma around neck and lower jaw; abnormal facies with anteverted nostrils, short nose, mongoloid slant to eyes, tongue protruding. No palmar or digital creases evident. (**C**) Internally, the heart had a membranous ventricular septal defect with passage of the valve leaflet through the A-V canal. The gut was malrotated. The lungs, kidneys, ovaries and uterus, and other organ systems were normal.

Estimated developmental age: 13 weeks
Fertilization age: 14 weeks
Karyotype: 47,XX,+22

# CHAPTER 5

# Tetraploidy

Tetraploidy is a relatively rare finding among spontaneous abortions and occurred in a total of 65 specimens examined morphologically. The interpretation of tetraploidy in a cultured specimen is always open to question, because tetraploidization is a common event in cultured cells, especially in cells from trophoblast or membrane, and in slowly growing cultures. Thus it is likely that some specimens classified as tetraploid actually were diploid but became tetraploid in vitro. This is borne out by a study in which we compared chromosome preparations from uncultured trophoblastic cells in chorionic villi with those from cultured cells. In two out of 37 cases studied, direct preparations were diploid, but cultured preparations were tetraploid (Yu et al., 1987). Cases in the study reported here were classified as tetraploid only if no diploid cells were observed in the 10 cells examined. The sex chromosome constitution was XXXX in 39 cases and XXYY in 26 cases.

## Distribution of Specimen Classes

Table 5-1 shows the distribution of specimens classes among tetraploid specimens. There were two specimens that were fetuses over 30 mm in length and one that was a well-formed embryo. The two fetuses were both without detectable malformation, but were autolyzed specimens retained in utero after fetal death. One was of 17-weeks gestation and 9-weeks developmental age; the other was of 25-weeks gestation and 21-weeks develop-

**Table 5-1** Morphological Class Among Tetraploid Specimens

|  | Number | % of Complete Specimens |
|---|---|---|
| Fragment | 28 | — |
| Intact empty sac | 28 | 75.7 |
| Small disorganized embryo (1–10 mm) | 6 | 16.2 |
| Sac with cord, embryo missing or fragment | 0 | 0 |
| Embryo or part of embryo (≤30 mm) | 1 | 2.7 |
| Fetus | 2 | 5.4 |
| Total cases examined | 65 |  |

mental age. Karyotype analysis was successful in both cases only from placental tissue. Thus it is possible that the tetraploidy is an artefact of culture.

The embryo was well preserved with a fertilization age of 46 days and a developmental age estimated at 35 days (Fig. 5–5). No abnormalities were noted, but again the karyotype was derived from culture of placental membranes and villi.

All other specimens were either placental fragments (43%), small disorganized embryos (9%), or intact empty sacs (43%) (Figs. 5–2 through 5–4). Among complete tetraploid specimens the proportion of intact empty sacs (76%) was the highest for any karyotype group: trisomy 16 had the next highest proportion (47%) of this specimen class.

## Gestational Age at Abortion

Tetraploid specimens had a mean gestational age of 12 weeks, similar to that for trisomy 16 and the nonviable trisomies. Apart from the two specimens which were large fetuses, there were 10 pregnancies with gestations reported beyond 13 weeks of age, including an intact empty sac reported as 22-weeks gestation. This might represent an error in dating the pregnancy by LMP, or extremely long retention of a conception with rudimentary development.

## Maternal Age

The mean maternal age of tetraploid pregnancies was 26.0, which is not different from that for triploid spontaneous abortions or livebirths in the same institution. There is no evidence for an effect of maternal age on the frequency of tetraploidy.

## Chorionic Villi

Only 16 tetraploid specimens had villi examined morphologically: the small proportion is due to the lack of observable villi in many specimens. Seventy-five percent of specimens had villi classified as normal. The lack of an association with cystic villi or hydatidiform mole in these polyploid specimens is in agreement with previous studies. Only in rare specimens arising from trispermy, with three paternal complements, have hydatidiform changes been observed (Sheppard et al., 1982; Surti et al., 1986).

## Discussion

Although it is likely that some cases classified as tetraploid are due to artefacts of culture, several lines of evidence suggest that tetraploid postimplantation conceptions exist.

First, the overall frequency of tetraploid specimens (approximately 3%) is quite similar among all studies of spontaneous abortions, arguing against a cultural phenomenon which might be expected to vary among laboratories using differing techniques of culture and analysis. Second, one specimen type, the intact empty sac, predominates among all studies (Carr, 1971; Creasy et al., 1976; Lauritsen, 1976; Boué et al., 1976), suggesting that there is a real entity being identified by this karyotype. Among our specimens there was one case of a twin pregnancy with two empty sacs. Although cultured separately, each was completely tetraploid upon analysis. Another possible interpretation is that the tissue from an empty sac is particularly likely to undergo tetraploidization in culture.

Tetraploid karyotypes, usually mosaic but occasionally apparently nonmosaic, have also been rarely reported among livebirths or prenatal diagnoses with multiple congenital anomalies (Golbus et al., 1976; Pitt et al., 1980; Veneema et al., 1982; Scarbrough et al., 1984; Shiono et al., 1988; Lafer et al., 1988). Here too there is sometimes the possibility of cultural artefact or tissue mosaicism.

In all studies to date, the XXXX set chromosome complement has been more frequent than the XXYY type. This may reflect growth of maternal cells that became tetraploid in some poorly growing cultures, or some increased survival rate for XXXX conceptions.

Although it is theoretically possible that tetraploid conceptions could arise through fusion of two diploid gametes, this does not appear to be the mechanism for those that have been observed. In almost all cases to date with an XXXX or XXYY sex chromosome complement, analysis of chromosome polymorphisms has shown that there appears to be two identical chromosome sets derived from an originally diploid zygote. Thus the tetraploidy arose as a result of failure of the first or a very early mitotic division of the zygote. Very rare cases of tetraploid conceptions with an XXXY sex chromosome complement have been described and shown to result from trispermy (Sheppard et al., 1982; Surti et al., 1986).

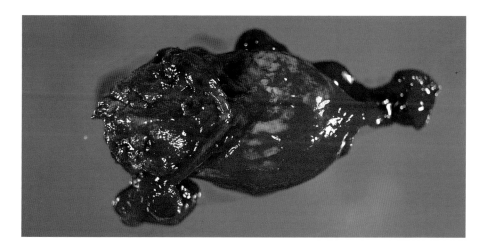

**Figure 5–1** (2480) Uterine cast covered by smooth maternal decidua: blood clot attached to upper margin, extending to the right (the cervical end?); villi and hemorrhage on left. The cast contained a 15-mm ruptured amnion and an amorphous embryo in two fragments measuring less than 2 mm.

Fertilization age: 11 weeks
      Karyotype: 92,XXXX

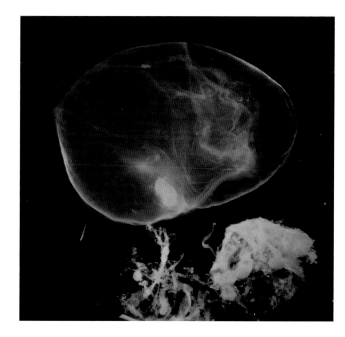

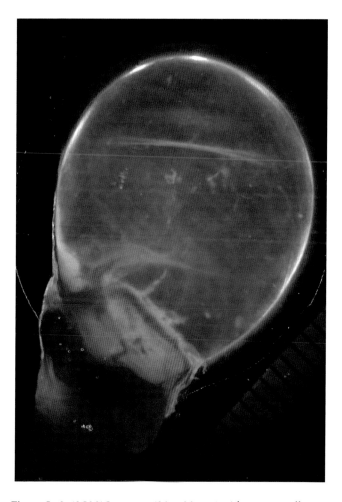

**Figure 5–2** (3530) Intact sac containing a 2-mm CRL embryo attached directly to the amnion.

Fertilization age: 10 weeks
      Karyotype: 92,XXXX

**Figure 5–3** (2500) Intact sac (20 × 20 mm) with a very small area of attachment to the placenta at lower end. A 1-mm CRL embryo (not seen in this picture) attached directly to amnion.

Fertilization age: 9 weeks
      Karyotype: 92,XXXX

**Figure 5–4** (2406) Intact sac (20 × 20 mm) entirely free of villi, or maternal tissue. A 3-mm CRL amorphous embryo found among the hemorrhagic tissue seen at one end.

Fertilization age: unknown
    Karyotype: 92,XXYY

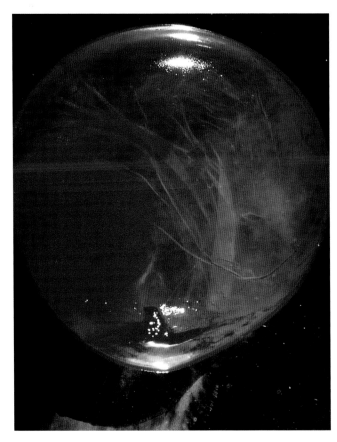

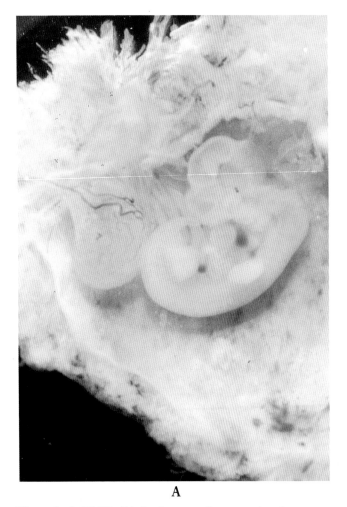

**A**

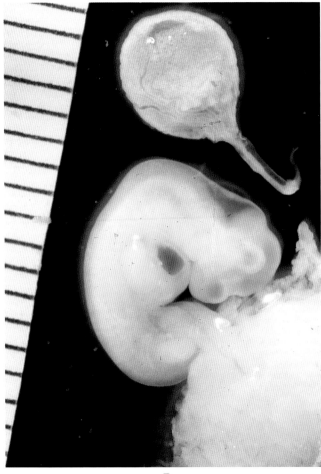

**Figure 5–5** (1952) (**A**) An 8-mm well-preserved embryo contained within a 10-mm intact amnion, within a 35-mm intact chorion that is entirely covered with villi. Upper and lower limb buds visible. (**B**) Blood filled heart prominence, somites and cephalic vesicles, vascular yolk sac, and cord with three vessels also visible.

Estimated developmental age: 35 days
    Fertilization age: 60 days
        Karyotype: 92,XXXX

**B**

# References

Angell RR, Templeton AA, Aitken RJ. 1986. Chromosome studies in human in vitro fertilization. Hum Genet 72:333–339.

Benacerraf B, Gelman R, Frigoletto FD. 1987. Sonographic identification of second-trimester fetuses with Down's syndrome. New Engl J Med 317:1371–1376.

Boué A, Boué J. Les arrêts du développement. 1980. In: Boué A, Henrion R, David G (eds.). Développement Prénatal Normal et Pathologique. Paris, Flammarion, pp. 449–476.

Boué A, Boué J, Gropp A. 1985. Cytogenetics of pregnancy wastage. Adv Hum Genet 14:1–57.

Boué J, Boué A. 1973. Anomalies chromosomiques dans las avortements spontanés. In: Boué A, Thibault C (eds.). Les Accidents Chromosomiques de la Reproduction. Paris, INSERM, pp. 29–55.

Boué J, Philippe E, Giroud A, Boué A. 1976. Phenotypic expression of lethal chromosomal anomalies in human abortuses. Teratology 14:3–20.

Brandriff B, Gordon L, Ashworth L, Watchmaker G, Moore D, Wyrobek AJ, Carrano AV. 1985. Chromosomes of human sperm: Variability among normal individuals. Hum Genet 70:18–24.

Byrne J. 1983. Fetal Pathology Laboratory Manual. Birth Defects Original Article Series, 19(2).

Byrne J, Blanc WA. 1985. Malformations and chromosome anomalies in spontaneously aborted fetuses with single umbilical artery. Am J Ob Gyn 151:340–342.

Byrne J, Blanc WA, Warburton D, Wigger J. 1984. The significance of cystic hygromata in fetuses. Hum Pathol 15:61–67.

Byrne, J, Warburton, D. 1979. Some pathological observations in spontaneous abortion. Birth Defects Original Article Series Vol XV No 5A:127–136.

Byrne J, Warburton, D. 1986. Neural tube defects in spontaneous abortion. Am J Med Genet 25:327–333.

Byrne J, Warburton D, Kline J, Blanc W, Stein Z. 1985. Morphology of early fetal deaths and their chromosomal characteristics. Teratology 32:297–315.

Canki N, Warburton D, Byrne J. 1988. Morphological characteristics of monosomy X in spontaneous abortion. Ann Génét 31:4–13.

Carr DH. 1967. Chromosome anomalies as a cause of spontaneous abortion. Am J Ob Gyn 97:283–293.

Carr DH, Gideon M. 1971. Chromosome studies in selected spontaneous abortions: Polyploidy in man. J Med Genet 8:1264–1274.

Chervenak FA, Isaacson G, Blakemore KJ, Breg WR, Hobbins JC, Berkowitz KG, Totora K, Mayden K, Mahoney MJ. 1983. Fetal cystic hygroma: Cause and natural history. N Eng J Med 309:822–825.

Creasy MR. 1976. Triploidy. Dev Med Ch Neurol 18:811–816.

Creasy MR, Crolla JA, Alberman EA. 1976. A cytogenetic study of human spontaneous abortions using banding techniques. Hum Genet 31:177–196.

Geisler M, Kleinebrecht J. 1978. Cytogenetic and histologic analyses of spontaneous abortions. Hum Genet 45:239–251.

Golbus MS, Bachman R, Wiltse S, Hall BD. 1976. Tetraploidy in a newborn infant. J Med Genet 13:329–332.

Graham JM, Rawnsley EF, Simmons GM, Wurster-Hill DH, Park JP, Maria-Radilla M, Crow HC. 1989. Triploidy: Pregnancy complications and clinical findings in seven cases. Prenatal Diagnosis 9:409–420.

Gullotta F, Rehder H, Gropp A. 1981. Descriptive neuropathology of chromosomal disorders in man. Hum Genet 57:337–344.

Harris MJ, Poland BJ, Dill FJ. 1981. Triploidy in 40 human spontaneous abortuses: assessment of phenotype in embryos. Obstet Gynecol 57:600–606.

Hassold T, Chen N, Funkhouser J, Jooss T, Manuel B, Matsuura J, Matsuyama A, Wilson C, Yamane JA, Jacobs PA. 1980. A cytogenetic study of 1000 spontaneous abortions. Ann Hum Genet 44:151–178.

Hassold T, Benham F, Leppert M. 1988. Cytogenetic and molecular analysis of sex-chromosome monosomy. Am J Hum Genet 42:534–541.

Hecht F, Macfarlane JP. 1969. Mosaicism in Turner's syndrome. Lancet 2:1197.

Hoagland MH, Frank KA, Hutchins GM. 1988. Prune belly syndrome with prostatic hypoplasia, bladder wall rupture, and massive ascites in a fetus with trisomy 18. Arch Pathol Lab Med 112:1126–1128.

Honoré LH, Dill FJ, Poland BJ. 1976. Placental morphology in spontaneous abortuses with normal and abnormal karyotypes. Teratology 14:151–166.

Hook E, Warburton D. 1983. The distribution of chromosomal genotypes associated with Turner's syndrome: livebirth prevalence rates and evidence for diminished fetal mortality and severity in genotypes associated with structural X abnormalities or mosaicism. Hum Genet 64:24–27.

Hunt PA, Jacobs PA, Szulman AE. 1983. Molar pregnancies and non-molar triploids; results of a 7-year cytogenetic study. Am J Hum Genet 35:135A.

Jacobs P, Hassold T. 1980. The origin of chromosome abnormalities in spontaneous abortion. In: Porter IH, Hook EB (eds.). Human Embryonic and Fetal Death. New York, Academic Press, pp. 289–298.

Jacobs PA, Szulman AE, Funkhouser J, Matsuura JS, Wilson CC. 1982. Human triploidy: Relationship between parental origin of the additional haploid complement and development of partial hydatidiform mole. Ann Hum Genet 46:223–231.

Kajii T, Ohama K, Niikawa N, Ferrier A, Avirachan S. 1973. Banding analyses of abnormal karyotypes in spontaneous abortion. Am J Hum Genet 25:539–547.

Kajii T, Ohama K. 1979. Inverse maternal age effect in monosomy X. Hum Genet 51:147–151.

Kinoshita M, Nakamura Y, Nakano R, Morimatsu M, Fukuda S, Nishimi Y, Hashimoto T. 1989. Thirty-one autopsy cases of Trisomy 18: Clinical features and pathological findings. Ped Path 9:445–457.

Kleinebrecht J, Geisler M. 1975. Histological analysis of spontaneous abortions with trisomy 2: First description of an embryo. Humangenetik 29:15–22.

Kleinebrecht J, Geisler M. 1984. Embryos with chromosomal aberrations from spontaneous abortions. Anat Anz Jena 157:3–33.

Kline J, Stein ZA. 1985. Environmental causes of aneuploidy: Why so elusive? In: Dellarco VL, Voytek PE, Hollaender A (eds.). Aneuploidy: Etiology and Mechanisms. New York, Plenum Press, pp. 149–164.

Lafer CZ, Neu RL. 1988. A liveborn infant with tetraploidy. Am J Med Genet 375:375–378.

Lauritsen JG. 1976. Aetiology of spontaneous abortion: A cytogenetic and epidemiological study of 288 abortuses and their parents. Acta Obstet Gyn Scand Suppl 52:1–29.

Lockwood C, Benacerraf B, Krinsky A, Blakemore K, Belanger K, Mahoney M, Hobbins J. 1987a. A sonographic screening method for Down syndrome. Am J Ob Gyn 157:803–808.

Lockwood C, Scioscia A, Stiller R, Hobbins J. 1987b. Sonographic features of the triploid fetus. Am J Ob Gyn 1577:285–287.

Martin RH, Rademaker AW. 1987. The effect of age on the frequency of sperm chromosomal abnormalities in normal men. Am J Hum Genet 41:484–492.

Martin RH, Rademaker AW, Hildebrand K, Long-Simpson L, Peterson D, Yamamoto J. 1987. Variations in the frequency and type of sperm chromosome abnormalities among normal men. Hum Genet 77:108–114.

Maudlin I, Fraser LR. 1978. Maternal age and the incidence of aneuploidy in first-cleavage mouse embryos after in vitro fertilization. J Reprod Fert 54:423–426.

Minguillon C, Eiben B, Bahr-Porsch S, Vogel M, Hansmann I. 1989. The predictive value of chorionic villus histology for identifying chromosomally normal and abnormal spontaneous abortions. Hum Genet 82:373–376.

Moerman P, Fryns JP, van der Steen K, Kleczkowska A, Lauweryns J. 1988. The pathology of Trisomy 13 syndrome: A study of 12 cases. Hum Genet 80:349–356.

Moore KL. 1988. The Developing Human (4th ed.). Philadelphia, WB Saunders.

Morton NE, Chiu D, Holland C, Jacobs PA, Pettay D. 1987. Chromosome anomalies as predictors of recurrence risk for spontaneous abortion. Am J Med Genet 28:353–360.

Nishimura H. 1983. Atlas of Human Prenatal Histology. Tokyo, Igaku-Shoin.

Nishimura H, Okamoto N. 1976. Sequential Atlas of Human Congenital Malformations. Tokyo, Igaku-Shoin.

Ohama K, Kusumi I, Ihara T. 1977. Trisomy 17 in two abortuses. Jap J Hum Genet 21:257–260.

O'Rahilly R, Muller F. 1987. Developmental Stages in Human Embryos. Publication 637, Carnegie Institution of Washington.

Pellestor F, Selè B. 1988. Assessment of aneuploidy in the human female by using cytogenetics of IVF failures. Am J Hum Genet 42:274–283.

Penrose LS, Delhanty JD. 1961. Triploid cell cultures from a macerated foetus. Lancet 1:1261–1262.

Peters MT, Lockwood CJ, Miller WA. 1989. The efficacy of fetal sonographic biometry in Down Syndrome screening. Am J Ob Gyn 161:297–300.

Philippe E. 1973. Morphologie et morphometric des placentas d'aberration chromosomique léthale. Rev Fr Gyn Obstet 68:645–649.

Philippe E, Boué JG. 1969. Le placenta des aberrations chromosomiques léthales. Ann Anat Path (Paris) 14:249–266.

Philippe E, Boué J, Boué A. 1980. Les maladies trophoblastiques gestationnelles. Ann Anat Path (Paris) 25:13–38.

Pitt D, Leversha M, Sinfield C, Campbell P, Anderson R, Bryan D, Rogers J. 1980. Tetraploidy in a liveborn infant with spina bifida and other anomalies. J Med Genet 18:309–311.

Poland BJ, Miller JR. 1973. Effect of karyotype in zygotic development. In: Boué A, Thibault C (eds.). Les Accidents Chromosomiques de la Reproduction. Paris, INSERM, pp. 111–118.

Poland BJ, Miller JR, Jones D, Trimble BK. 1977. Reproductive counseling in patients who had a spontaneous abortion. Am J Ob Gyn 127:685–691.

Putte van der SCJ. 1977. Lymphatic malformation in human fetuses. V Arch A Path Anat Histol 376:233–246.

Rehder H, Coerdt W, Eggers R, Klink F, Schwinder E. 1989. Is there any correlation between morphological and cytogenetic findings in placental tissue from early missed abortions? Hum Genet 82:377–385.

Reik W. 1989. Genomic imprinting and genetic disorders in man. Trends in Genetics 5(10):331–336.

Sanger R, Tippet P, Gavin J, Teesdale P, Daniels GL. 1977. Xg groups and sex chromosome abnormalities in people of northern European ancestry: An addendum. J Med Genet 14:210–213.

Scarbrough PR, Hersh J, Kukolich MK, Carroll AJ, Finley SC,

Hochberger R, Wilkerson S, Yen FF, Althaus BW. 1984. Tetraploidy: a report of three liveborn infants. Am J Med Genet 19:29–37.

Schinzel A. 1984. Catalogue of Unbalanced Chromosome Aberrations in Man. New York, WG de Gruyter.

Sheppard DM, Fisher RA, Lawler SD, Povey S. 1982. Tetraploid conceptus with three paternal contributions. Hum Genet 62:371–374.

Sheppard TH, Wener MH, Myhre SA, Hickok DE. 1986. Lowered serum albumin in fetal Turner's syndrome. J Pediat 108:114–116.

Shiono H, Azumi J, Fukiwara M, Wamazaki H, Kikuchi. 1988. Tetraploidy in a 15-month-old girl. Am J Med Genet 29:543–547.

Singh RP, Carr DH. 1966. The anatomy and histology of XO human embryos and fetuses. Anat Rec 155:369–381.

Sperber GH, Honore LM, Machin GA. 1989. Microscopic study of holoprosencephalic facial anomalies in Trisomy 13 fetuses. Am J Med Genet 32:443–451.

Surti U, Szulman AE, Wagner K, Leppert M, O'Brien SJ. 1986. Tetraploid partial hydatidiform moles: two cases with a triple paternal contribution and an XXXY karyotype. Hum Genet 72:15–21.

Takahara H, Ohama K, Fujiwara A. 1977. Cytogenetic study in early spontaneous abortion. Hiroshima J Med Sci 26:291–296.

Uchida IA, Freeman VCP. 1985. Triploidy and chromosomes. Am J Ob Gyn 151:65–69.

Veneema H, Tasseron EWK. 1982. Mosaic tetraploidy in a male neonate. Clin Genet 19:295–298.

Warburton D. 1987. Reproductive loss: How much is preventable? N Engl J Med 36:158–160.

Warburton D, Fraser FC. 1964. Spontaneous abortion risks in man: data from reproductive histories collected in a medical genetics unit. Am J Hum Genet 16:1–24.

Warburton D, Kline J, Stein Z, Hutzler M, Chin A, Hassold T. 1987. Does the karyotype of a spontaneous abortion predict the karyotype of a subsequent abortion? Evidence from 273 women with two karyotyped spontaneous abortions. Am J Hum Genet 41:465–483.

Warburton D, Kline J, Stein ZA, Strobino B. 1986. Cytogenetic abnormalities in spontaneous abortions of recognized conceptions. In: Porter IH, Hatcher NH, Willey AM (eds.). Perinatal Genetics: Diagnosis and Treatment. New York, Academic Press, pp. 23–40.

Warburton D, Kline J, Stein Z, Susser M. 1980. Monosomy X:

a chromosomal anomaly associated with young maternal age. Lancet: 1:167–169.

Warburton D, Stein Z, Kline J, Susser M. 1980. Chromosome abnormalities in spontaneous abortions: Data from the New York study. In: Porter IH, Hook EB (eds.). Human Embryonic and Fetal Death, New York, Academic Press, pp. 261–287.

Warburton D, Strobino B. 1987. Recurrent spontaneous abortion. In: Bennet MJ, Edmonds DK (eds.). Spontaneous and Recurrent Abortion, Oxford, Blackwell Scientific Publications, pp. 193–213.

Watt JL, Templeton AA, Messinis I, Bell L, Cunningham P, Duncan RO. 1987. Trisomy 1 in an eight cell human embryo. J Med Genet 24:60–64.

Wilcox AJ, Weinberg CR, O'Connor JF, Baird DD, Schlalterer JP, Canfield RE, Armstrong EG, Nisula BC. 1988. Incidence of early loss of pregnancy. N Eng J Med 319:189–194.

Wramsby H, Fredga K, Liedholm P. 1987. Chromosome analysis of human oocytes recovered from preovulatory follicles in stimulated cycles. N Eng J Med 316:121–124.

Yu MT, Warburton D, Yu C-Y. 1987. Direct chorionic villus preparations for karyotyping spontaneous abortions. Am J Hum Genet 41: Abstract

Zerres K, Niesen M, Schwanitz G, Hansmann M. 1988. Trisomy 22—prenatal findings in various developmental stages. Geburtschilfe Frauenheilkd 48:720–723.

# Index

Abdomen, 53, 90. *See also* Prune belly
Abortion
  elective, 3, 6, 61, 70, 72
  missed, 9, 37
  spontaneous, 3, 5
    chromosome anomalies in, 3, 4, 39
    definition, 5
    early, 3
    frequency, 3, 9, 57
    recurrence of, 4
    women in sample, 5
Adrenals
  hypoplastic, 37, 52, 54, 56, 58, 60, 65, 70
  normal, 84
Age. *See* Developmental age; Fertilization age; Gestational
    age; Maternal age; Paternal age
Amnion, 64, 73, 76–79. *See also* Sac
Anencephaly. *See* Brain
Aorta
  coarctation, 18, 20, 28, 30
  descending, 28, 65, 81
Artery
  carotid, 30, 70
  internal iliac, 32
  intersegmental, 32
  pulmonary, 28
  subclavian, 32
  umbilical, single, 18, 28, 31, 32, 43, 53, 54, 65, 82, 85
Ascites, 18
Auricular hillocks, *See* Ear
Autolysis, 9, 12
  in monosomy X, 19, 20
  in triploidy, 37

Bladder, 32, 84
Body stalk, 47, 74
Brain, *See also* Hydrocephaly, Neural tube defects
  forebrain, 74

malformations
  anencephaly, 47, 61
  cyclocephaly, 39, 60
  encephalocele, 19, 24, 26, 61, 74
  exencephaly, 87
  macrocephaly, 85
  microcephaly, 40
Brown bumps. *See* Hemorrhage

Cervical flexure, 22, 25, 26, 45, 74
Chorionic villi. *See* villi
Cleft lip, 60, 61, 69, 80, 82, 87
Cleft palate, 9, 58, 60, 61, 65, 69, 82
  physiological, 24, 26, 27, 91
Clubbed feet, *See* Feet, talipes
Colobomata. *See* Eye
Cord
  dilated, 18, 19, 24, 26, 43, 47, 75, 76, 87
  short, 88
  thin, 52–54
  twisted, 51, 88
  umbilical, 9, 18, 21, 22, 32, 43, 46, 47, 56, 58, 75–77,
    87, 88, 91
  vessels, 21, 96. *See also* Artery, single umbilical; Veins,
    umbilical
Cranial vault, 47
Crown-rump length (CRL), 12, 39

Demographics, study population, 6
Development
  arrested, 39
  asynchronous, 9, 12, 22, 25, 27, 40, 46, 68, 91
  retarded, 9, 12, 25, 37, 40
  timetables, 12, 12–13*f*, 39
Developmental age, 5, 9, 37
Digits. *See also* Feet
  abnormal position, 83
  absent flexion creases, 84, 92

Italic letter *f* following an arabic number denotes a figure; italic letter *t* indicates a table.

101